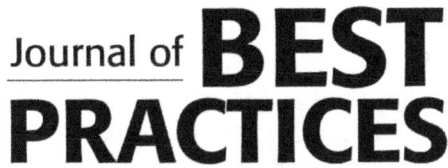

Journal of **BEST PRACTICES**
in **Health Professions Diversity:**
Research, Education, and Policy

W0038150

SPRING 2024

Founded in 2007, *The Journal of Best Practices in Health Professions Diversity* (ISSN 2475-2843) is published by the University of North Carolina Press for the School of Health Sciences at Winston-Salem State University. Directed toward educators, policymakers, and the health community, it is a source of peer-reviewed information on maximizing recruitment and retention of culturally diverse students for careers in the health professions.

Submissions

All manuscripts should conform to the *Publication Manual of the American Psychological Association* (7th ed.) with respect to format, style, grammar, punctuation, mechanics, and citation. They should be prepared for blind review. Authors are asked to submit an electronic version of manuscripts in Microsoft Word or ASCII text. Manuscripts may be submitted via email to walkerq@wssu.edu, or via mail to:

Quiteya D. Walker, PhD, LCMHCA, NCC, CRC, Managing Editor
Journal of Best Practices in Health Professions Diversity
School of Health Sciences
241 F.L. Atkins Building
Winston-Salem State University
601 S. Martin Luther King Jr. Drive
Winston-Salem, NC 27110

Articles will be selected upon review and recommendation by the editorial board. The board may request additional information and editing. Articles will be evaluated for writing style and readability, logical development, methodology, and appropriateness to the stated subject matter of the journal. All manuscripts will be returned. Authors should expect to be informed of publication status approximately one month prior to publication.

The Journal of Best Practices in Health Professions Diversity is included in JSTOR's Public Health Collection. It is also available digitally from EBSCO and ProQuest. Print subscriptions are not available, but print copies of each issue can be purchased from UNC Press. Please visit https://uncpress.org/journals/journal-of-best-practices-in-health-professions-diversity/ for more information.

JOURNAL OF BEST PRACTICES IN HEALTH PROFESSIONS DIVERSITY:
RESEARCH, EDUCATION, AND POLICY

Volume 17 • Number 1 • Spring 2024

Table of Contents

Diverse Perspectives in Healthcare Education: A Call for Thoughtful Integration

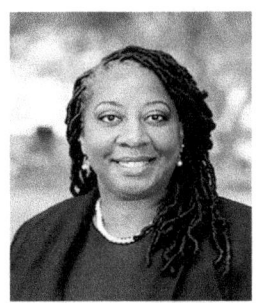

In the evolving landscape of healthcare education, the integration of diverse perspectives and cultural awareness has become increasingly important. The articles presented in this issue of the *Journal of Best Practices in Health Professions Diversity* collectively highlight the necessity for healthcare curricula to thoughtfully engage with these concepts.

As demographic shifts continue to reshape the patient population, healthcare professionals must be equipped with the knowledge and skills to deliver care that is responsive to the varied backgrounds of the communities they serve. This issue explores various aspects of this educational imperative, addressing both the challenges and opportunities that arise in current practices.

Research by Brown et al. sheds light on gaps in healthcare education programs' assessment of competencies related to cultural awareness. Despite recognizing their importance, many assessments do not explicitly measure the relevant knowledge, skills, and behaviors. This oversight may limit the preparation of future healthcare providers who can effectively meet the needs of a diverse patient population.

The article by Mazurek emphasizes the significance of cultivating a workforce that reflects anticipated demographic changes in the coming decades. A well-prepared workforce can enhance the relevance of care delivered to various communities. This article advocates for thoughtful changes in recruitment, training, and retention practices to create a more inclusive educational environment.

The perspectives shared by Sherrod and Daniels provide valuable insights into the experiences of students navigating healthcare education. Their narratives underscore the importance of supportive environments that foster a sense of belonging, ultimately contributing to a more effective learning experience. By amplifying these voices, we can better understand the barriers that exist and the strategies that can be employed to address them.

The contributions in this issue collectively encourage stakeholders in healthcare education to consider how curricula and assessments can be aligned with the diverse needs of the workforce and patient populations. Ensuring that educational practices meet these needs is critical for preparing healthcare professionals to provide high-quality care in a variety of settings.

Looking ahead, educational institutions, policymakers, and healthcare organizations must work together to create a cohesive approach to training. This collaborative effort will enhance the competency of healthcare providers and contribute to improved health outcomes across communities.

In conclusion, the articles in this issue serve as a reminder of the ongoing need for thoughtful engagement with diverse perspectives in healthcare education. By focusing on the continuous assessment and enhancement of educational practices, we can shape a healthcare workforce that is knowledgeable, empathetic, and capable of addressing the varied needs of the populations they serve. We invite readers to engage with this critical discourse and reflect on the role they can play in fostering an effective and responsive healthcare system.

Leslee Battle, EdD

Leslee Battle

Editor-in-Chief

Dismantling the Barriers to Health Professions Diversity

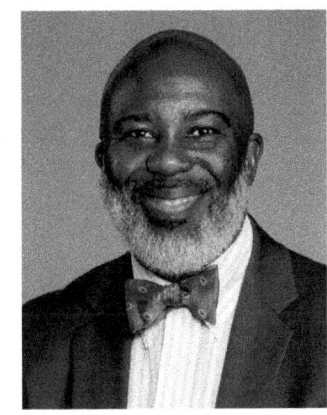

The recent attacks on diversity, equity, and inclusion in education have made the rapidly approaching election of a new president critical. The words of former NAMME President Dr. Anika Daniels-Osaze proved prophetic when she posited that healthcare and diversity would be challenged. Unfortunately, she predicted the SCOTUS decision on affirmative action in college admissions. The dismantling of policies and re-allocation, reduction, or, in some instances, elimination of funding for critical programs has put the development and sustainability of a diverse health professions workforce in peril. As health scientists and educators, we must think outside the box and marshal all of our resources to ensure that the next generation of health professionals become increasingly diverse and representative of the populations they serve.

Former HHS Secretary Dr. Louis W. Sullivan declared that increasing the diversity of the health professions would improve access to high-quality healthcare for minority patients, assuring a sound healthcare system for all. He knew that strengthening healthcare delivery systems would enhance educational experiences for all health professions students and promote relevant research and much-needed changes in our health policies, which, in turn, would prepare our nation for the emerging, culturally dynamic challenges to come (Sullivan Alliance, 2004, p.13).

The National Association of Medical Minority Educators, Inc. (NAMME), founded in 1975 on the campus of Howard University, has been at the forefront in addressing the concerns and mechanisms to ensure access to health professions training programs. Its initial focus was the shortage of minority physicians. Now, its mission includes all health professions programs.

This year, NAMME held its national conference and recruitment fair in Chicago, Illinois. Our theme was "Staying the Course: Protecting Diversity, Equity, and Inclusion." Our time was spent listening to educators promote DEI in medical education, while warning about the damaging consequences of some states' policy changes. As educators, researchers, and policymakers, we must share our knowledge and best practices for increasing the diversity of the health professions.

The missions of the *Journal of Best Practices in Health Professions Diversity* and NAMME are perfectly aligned, and the articles in this journal reflect it. Every topic is timely and should be consulted and cited when working to level the playing field for the next generation of health professionals.

REFERENCE

Sullivan Alliance. (2004). *Sullivan commission report on health professions diversity.* Washington, DC: National Academies Press.

Bernard M. Roper, PhD

President, National Association of Medical Minority Educators (NAMME)

ORIGINAL RESEARCH

Preparatory Program for Students Underrepresented in Medicine Promotes Self-Efficacy in the Medical School Application Process: Novel Insights from a Qualitative Analysis

Brian Zenger, MD, PhD[1,4]; Allison Chang, MD[3]; Donna Rae Eldridge, MSW[1]; Sofia Pauline Thoms[2]; Yvannia Marie Gray[2]; Ashley Kang, BSc[2]; Benjamin A. Steinberg, MD, MHS[1]; T. Jared Bunch, MD[1]; Akiko Kamimura, PhD[2]; Line Kemeyou, MD[1]; Paloma F. Cariello, MD, MPH[1]

Author Affiliations: [1]University of Utah School of Medicine, Salt Lake City, Utah; [2]University of Utah College of Social Work, University of Utah, Salt Lake City, Utah; [3]John A. Burns School of Medicine (JABSOM), University of Hawaii, Honolulu, Hawaii; [4]Washington University School of Medicine, St. Louis, Missouri

Corresponding Author: Brian Zenger, University of Utah Health Sciences Center, 30 North 1900 East, Salt Lake City, UT 84132 (*brian.zenger@hsc.utah.edu*)

ABSTRACT

Background: The current US physician workforce does not reflect the diversity of the patient population it serves. While programs have been designed to support learners underrepresented in medicine, evidence of their efficacy is lacking. **Methods:** We designed, implemented, and assessed a medical school admissions preparatory program (MAPP) for premedical students from underrepresented backgrounds, as defined by race, gender identity, and/or socioeconomic status. The program includes workshops, near-peer mentorship, and professional standardized test-preparation materials. We assessed the students' development using a mixed-methods, post-test approach that included surveys and one-on-one interviews. Questions were based on social cognitive career theory. We used independent thematic

J Best Pract Health Prof Divers, (Spring, 2024), 17(1), 1–17.
ISBN 2745-2843 © Winston-Salem State University

analysis to extract key themes across interviews. **Results:** We surveyed and interviewed 13 of 17 MAPP participants in 2021. The cohort had a mean age of 23.7+/-4; 77% were women; and 23% self-identified as Asian, 15% as Pacific Islander, 15% as Black, 31% as Hispanic, and 23% as American Indian. We found they had little experience with the medical school application process and developed new insights about themselves from participating in MAPP. The primary drivers of growth were (1) guidance in the medical school admission process, (2) near-peer mentorship and interactions, and (3) sense of community with other program participants. **Conclusion:** MAPP provided materials and methods that clarified the process and bolstered students' confidence in their ability to complete the application.

Keywords: ▪ Diversity ▪ Diversity in Medicine ▪ Medical School Admissions ▪ Qualitative Analysis ▪ Racial Justice

Authors' Note: Support for this research came from NIH NHLBI grant no. 1F30HL149327 (B.Z.) and K23HL143156 (B.A.S.), and NIH NCATS grant no. UL1TR002538 (RedCap Database UofU). B.A.S. reports research support from AHA/PCORI, Abbott, Cardiva, and AltaThera, and he consults for Sanofi and AltaThera. All other authors have no disclosures.

INTRODUCTION

The medical provider workforce lacks the diversity needed to properly care for the ever-more-diverse US patient population (AAMC, 2020; AHRQ, 2017; Aibana et al., 2019; Silver et al., 2019). Studies consistently show that most US physicians identify as Caucasian, cis-gendered, with a high socioeconomic status, despite significant patient populations identifying differently (AAMC, 2020; AHRQ, 2017; US Census Bureau, 2020). Of medical graduates in 2019, only 5.3% identified as Hispanic, 6.2% as Black, and 0.2% as Native American (AAMC, 2020), whereas 18.2% of the US population identifies as Hispanic, 12.2% as Black, and 0.6% as Native American (US Census Bureau, 2020). In addition to ethnic disparities, LGBTQ+, persons with disabilities, and low socioeconomic status groups are underrepresented in the physician workforce (AAMC, 2022; Grbic et al., 2015; Nouri et al., 2021; Youngclaus & Roskovensky, 2018).

Several studies show the importance of diverse healthcare teams (Alsan et al., 2019; Smedley et al., 2003). Patients who identify as underrepresented were more likely to seek care from providers of similar backgrounds and felt better supported by diverse care teams (Alsan et al., 2019; Takeshita et al., 2020). National professional societies acknowledge low diversity among physicians as a crucial systemic failure that must be addressed, yet ambitious plans for over two decades have achieved little progress (AAMC, 2020; Quality, 2017). In fact, the percentage of Black physicians has decreased over the past ten years (Talamantes et al., 2019).

Systemic failures occur even before potential physicians apply to medical school and continue through training and into careers (AHRQ, 2017; Smedley et al., 2003; Talamantes et al., 2019). This long, laborious process requires intense institutional or personal support, first, to complete the necessary premedical coursework and to achieve high GPAs and medical college admission test (MCAT) scores. Students must also demonstrate volunteer work, clinical exposure, shadowing, research, and leadership activities and produce strong recommendation letters from scholarly, research, and clinical mentors. They must compile this information into a coherent application that includes a personal statement and describes their activities. Beyond the application, they will be interviewed and must complete "secondary" applications. Finally, applying to each medical school incurs a fee, easily ballooning to thousands of dollars for each application cycle. Students from underrepresented backgrounds often lack the institutional support, mentorship, procedural knowledge, and financial resources to successfully apply to medical school in the United States.

Therefore, the application process is a good target for increasing diversity (AAMC, 2019). Numerous "premedical preparatory programs" have been developed and implemented throughout the United States (Campbell et al., 2014, 2022; Cantor et al., 1998; Keith & Hollar, 2012; Musick & Ray, 2015; Wrensford et al., 2019). They focus on teaching underrepresented students about standardized test preparation; ideal volunteer, leadership, and clinical experiences; and how to write a convincing personal statement and assemble the final application. Among the many approaches, the most common is a workshop series taught by content experts, such as admission committee members, medical school staff, or medical students (Keith & Hollar, 2012; Musick & Ray, 2015). Some programs include subscriptions to professional test-preparation resources, mentorship connections, or near-peer coaches (Cantor et al., 1998; Keith & Hollar, 2012).

Evaluation of these programs has mainly focused on such objective endpoints as medical school acceptance rates or interview invitations. While attesting to the success of individual programs, it does not capture whether and how they help students discover their passion for medicine or other career fields (Cantor et al., 1998; Keith & Hollar, 2012). Furthermore, the specific components that contribute to student growth are not identified. To improve these programs and clarify their impact, evaluations must determine precisely what students learn, what obstacles remain, and what changes can help to meet the needs of an ever-changing participant demographic.

Social cognitive career theory is a validated framework that can be applied to understand the impact of these preparatory programs. The theory delineates four categories of behavior—previous experience, self-efficacy, outcome expectations, and personal goal setting—that change as individuals feel more prepared, excited, motivated, and included in their respective careers (Lent et al., 2002). Here, we apply this framework to assess the impact of a medical school admissions preparatory program (MAPP) designed for students from backgrounds underrepresented in medicine. Our goal is to evaluate which components are most important and how they might be improved.

Our mixed-methods approach followed discrete surveys and one-on-one interviews with thematic analysis to identify all four social cognitive career categories.

METHODS

Preparatory Program Design and Procedure

Premedical students identified as underrepresented were encouraged to apply through various professional channels using web advertisements, social media outlets, email subscriptions, and direct contact with premedical advisors at local universities. Underrepresented status was defined by self-identified race and gender or sexual orientation; first generation in the family to attend higher education; or perceived low socioeconomic status. The 15-20 students accepted into the program annually anticipate applying to medical school within one-to-two years. Timing is the primary reason students could not participate; some were already applying to medical school, and others planned to apply two or more years after the program's start.

The Office of Health Equity, Diversity, and Inclusion (OHEDI) at the University of Utah School of Medicine launched the eight-week summer course and has enrolled students yearly since 2015.

The course has three main components: workshops, professional MCAT preparation materials, and near-peer mentoring. Weekly, one-hour workshops are led by teams of faculty, staff, and current medical students. Following the imposition of COVID-19 pandemic protections, they were conducted virtually via video conferencing. They address study techniques, the American Medical College Application Service (AMCAS) outline, financial aid, resumé building, and the personal statement and include practice interviews. Students also participated in an asynchronous MCAT preparation course purchased from Kaplan Test Preparation Services. Finally, students were randomly paired with a near-peer medical student mentor; matching was not based on background. They met at least once, and most met often; some stayed in touch after the program's conclusion. The OHEDI team selected the mentors before the year's MAPP began and financially compensated their service. The structure of the mentorship sessions was not specified. They varied from help with the personal statement to financial advice to life as a medical student (see https://medicine.utah.edu/ohedi/undergrad-premed/mcat-prep for further detail).

Sampling Strategy and Sample

All students who completed MAPP in 2021 were asked to participate in this study. The only criteria were completion of the program in 2021 and age 18 years and older. Students participated in an online survey and a virtual interview in March 2022 as detailed below.

Study Measures

The study was approved by the Institutional Review Board (Study ID:00150396). Before the interview, students were informed about the project and signed their consent to participate. They were then asked to complete an online survey consisting of 15 baseline demographic questions and establish whether they had previously participated in a medical school admissions preparatory course. Demographic questions included age, gender identity, race, and educational background (see Appendix 1). Data were acquired and stored in a secure online repository. No information from the student's MAPP application was included in this analysis.

One-on-One Interviews

Interview questions were based on social cognitive career theory, which provides a framework to evaluate the strengths and weaknesses of medical school admissions preparatory programs beyond strictly objective measures (Lent et al., 2002). Each student was asked 11 questions related to the theory's four categories: prior experience (3 questions), self-efficacy (5), outcome expectations (2), and personal goals (1). In the context of prospective medical students, previous experience includes any programs they had participated in and any relevant personal interactions. Self-efficacy refers to how students perceive their ability to apply to medical school and to craft a competitive application. Outcome expectations address specific actions; for example, what experiences do they believe will best support their application, or how do they deem their likelihood of acceptance. Personal goals explore whether and how the course enabled students to make their plans more specific and actionable; for example, does a goal change from "I want to get into medical school" to "I want to improve my MCAT score" or "to increase my shadowing experience" (see Table 1). Instrument design drew from instruments asking similar questions (Lent et al., 2002), but the literature offered no exact, validated match focusing on the assessment of MAPPs.

One member of the OHEDI team familiar with all program students conducted one-on-one virtual interviews. All interviews were recorded, transcribed, and stored on a secure server for analysis. They were completed over three weeks in March 2022.

Data Analysis

Data analysis was based on a thematic approach. Following the transcription of the interviews, two research assistants, who were not interviewers, performed initial coding and separately identified themes (Creswell & Creswell, 2017). A third research assistant resolved discrepancies between the two coders to select the best codes and examples and to ensure we achieved thematic saturation. We were able to forego member checking since the three research assistants had no relationship to the participants, were not involved in data collection, and were therefore unlikely to show bias. They all had qualitative research experience.

Table 1: Interview Questions by Social Cognitive Career Theory Category

Category	Question
Prior Experience	1. How prepared did you feel to apply to medical school prior to entering MAPP?
	2. Why did you decide to participate in MAPP?
	3. Prior to starting MAPP, how did you think it would help you to prepare to apply to medical school?
Self-efficacy	1. How did MAPP help you to understand the medical school application process?
	2. What components were most valuable in helping you to apply to medical school?
	3. How do you perceive yourself as a prospective applicant to medical school after completing MAPP?
	How did MAPP support you as a student from an underrepresented background?
	4. Do you feel there were any gaps in the MAPP experience?
Outcome Expectations	1. How has MAPP changed your ability to complete the medical school application process?
	2. How has MAPP changed your perspective on your potential to be accepted into medical school as a student from a diverse background?
Goals	1. How have your personal goals changed since completing MAPP?

Survey results for each study participant were collected from the electronic RedCap database. Responses to each question are displayed as number of students and percentage of the cohort. Since the survey had no open-ended questions, no thematic analysis was performed.

RESULTS

Thirteen students (76.5% of the total) were surveyed and interviewed approximately 8 months after completing MAPP. Those who did not participate in an interview did not make their reasons clear nor respond to several communications. Baseline demographic data and relevant educational background are also reported (see Table 2).

Table 2: Demographic and Educational Characteristics of Participants

Characteristics	Overall (n=13)
Age (mean (SD))	23.7 (4)
Gender (n (%))	
Male	2 (15%)
Female	10 (77%)
Nonbinary	1 (8%)
Race (n (%))	
White or Caucasian	1 (8%)
Asian	3 (23%)
Native Hawaiian or Pacific Islander	2 (15%)
Black or African American	2 (15%)
Hispanic or Latinx	4 (31%)
American Indian or Alaskan Native	3 (23%)
Expected College Graduation Year (n (%))	
2020	1 (8%)
2021	3 (23%)
2022	6 (46%)
2023	3 (23%)
College Major (n (%))	
Biology	3 (23%)
Human Biology	1 (8%)
Microbiology	1 (8%)
Kinesiology	1 (8%)
Psychology	1 (8%)
International Studies	1 (8%)
Physiological and Developmental Biology	1 (8%)

(Continued)

Table 2: *(Continued)*

Characteristics	Overall (n=13)
Recreational Therapy	1 (8%)
Business	1 (8%)
GPA *(mean (SD))*	3.5 (0.4)
Immediate Family Members Who Attended College (n (%))	
0	2 (15%)
1	3 (23%)
2	4 (31%)
5	4 (31%)

Prior Experience

Theme 1: Not prepared. Many of the students interviewed felt that they were not prepared to apply to medical school and attributed their lack of preparation to at least one of the components MAPP addresses. Some acknowledged that preparing for interviews were an area they had not considered. One stated, "I didn't feel very prepared at all to study for the MCAT or anything like that or didn't really know how to apply for medical school" [Participant A]. Another admitted, "I'd say not super-well prepared. I had done my own research, but I didn't know a lot of the specific details, especially when it came to ... the application itself and ... how the interviews would go" [Participant B].

Theme 2: Somewhat prepared. Other students commented on several areas in which they felt inadequate or underprepared. Many saw access to MCAT preparatory materials as critical. For example, one participant stated, "I didn't know a ton of the [admissions] processes that was talked about in the MAPP program, and I also really was struggling with ... preparing for the MCAT" [Participant C]. Another participant said:

> I'd say I felt maybe 60% prepared. I've ... received the list of extracurriculars and ... academic standings that medical program applications require of students and still felt like there were some pieces that I just maybe didn't have a lot of access to, like the physician shadowing or even materials for MCAT prep. [Participant D]

Based on our survey results, students had some experience in different areas relevant to their application before starting MAPP. All students (n=13, 100%) noted they had leadership, volunteer, and research experiences relevant to medical school applications. However, only six (46%) had previous experience with MCAT preparation, and only seven (54%) with physician shadowing.

Theme 3: No previous medical school admissions preparatory program experience. Based on the survey results, few students (n=3, 23%) had prior experience with medical school preparatory programs. They varied, but all targeted underrepresented students. At the time of the survey, only one student (8%) was enrolled in a preparatory program at another institution.

Self-Efficacy

Theme 1: More prepared after participating in MAPP. Many students felt more prepared to apply to medical school after MAPP. Most noted at least one of the main components as a reason and highlighted understanding the "application materials needed" and the "target MCAT score" depending on their situation. We discuss these contributing factors below.

Theme 2: More excited and confident. After the program, many students were more excited and confident about completing the medical school application process. Before, they noted negative feelings, including "imposter syndrome" (Clance & Imes, 1978). Students acknowledged feeling more "hope" and "self-worth" after completing MAPP.

Theme 3: More competitive. Students felt "more competitive" as a "worthy applicant" to medical school. They felt they would have more flexibility and could apply to, and be accepted by, more than one medical school.

MAPP Components that Increased Feelings of Self-Efficacy

Theme 1: Guidance into, and explanations about, the medical school process. Students related their increased feelings of self-efficacy to a clearer understanding of the admissions process. They noted that education about each component of the application was beneficial, including "how to get letters of recommendation," "how to talk about what you are doing in a way that's effective," "how to be holistic with the holistic review," and "pay attention to even small key points in my application." They acquired these insights from several sources, including the formal workshops, near-peer mentors, and OHEDI staff.

Theme 2: Near-peer mentors: Many students noted the effectiveness of working with near-peer medical student mentors throughout the MAPP and beyond. They pointed out that the mentors could "fill in questions that I had" beyond the formal education course. They also appreciated the longitudinal and personal connection with the mentorship team. One student stated:

> I loved being able to meet someone who was in medical school and helped guide me through the process because they've been through it, and they're able to, even now, still personally reach out and to check on me, and I check on them,

and I feel like that is the most valuable one of the most valuable things I took in the program. Because I can have that forever. [Participant F]

Theme 3: Community-building: The student community contributed significantly to self-efficacy. Students acknowledged the "encouragement" their peers provided. They felt connected at a deep level and have used those "connections" to "work together" to achieve a common "goal." One student remarked, "I feel it really helped me.... I was struggling with imposter syndrome, and honestly, seeing a lot of, I guess, minorities who were in ... the same position as me also really helped motivate me. It honestly gave me ... encouragement that I could" succeed [Participant G].

Outcome Expectations

Theme 1: More knowledgeable: Many students noted being more knowledgeable about the application process after completing MAPP. One reported:

> No one in my family has ever been to medical school—or close friends—and so that was ... a little ... frightening because I didn't know, like, what is this process?—you know, what do I need to do? But the program was awesome because ... learning about that was incredibly helpful. [Participant C]

Furthermore, students felt prepared to take on specific tasks of the application process. Knowing "what medical schools are looking for" gave them a feeling of satisfaction in completing the application, not just "like I was checking boxes."

Theme 2: Increased likelihood of acceptance: Many students felt they had a better chance of acceptance after completing MAPP. They noted that their increased understanding of the medical school admissions process gave them the tools for success. One stated:

> As a diverse student, I feel that my chances of getting into medical school have increased after the program because I know more about it. I know that the application is not heavily focused on just one area. Then it depends on how I present myself, and how well-rounded I am as an applicant, and it doesn't just rely on my GPA or MCAT score, which is heavily ... focused on in the premed environment. [Participant F]

Theme 3: Felt more qualified: Students also felt more qualified after completing MAPP. Specifically, one noted, I do not "consider myself an underdog anymore." MAPP helped students see that they were "valuable" and that their diversity was valuable in "all medical schools." They reconsidered their previous negative thoughts and focused on their positive abilities. After MAPP, they felt "capable of going to medical school now because, before the MAPP, I just didn't feel like I was good enough" [Participant A].

Personal Goals

Theme 1: Higher MCAT score goals: After participating in the MAPP, students had higher expectations and specific, actionable goals related to their MCAT performance. They commented that the resources MAPP provided gave them the tools necessary to succeed on the MCAT. One said, "I increased my goal for my MCAT, and so I know I could do better because of the MAPP. I have the resources to do better and that is a goal that I have improved on since the MAPP" [Participant F].

Theme 2: Being genuine in the application: Students noted a change in how they perceived the application. They focused on reflecting their character, not filling in a checklist based on earlier guidance or online resources. A student said, "One goal I did add was to really … focus more on what I have to offer, rather than trying to be that unique, stellar applicant. So that's one of my personal goals … really just … being who I am, embracing the fact of … who I am" [Participant H].

Theme 3: Focusing on self-care: Students commented on changing their approach to their own lives and ensuring they remain healthy and strong throughout the application process. They felt that the MAPP gave them the tools to be "more relaxed" and to spend more time "taking care of themselves." They noted that the knowledge, community, and mentorship provided by MAPP helped to alleviate the high stress of the medical school admissions process.

Areas for MAPP Improvement

Theme 1: Providing opportunities for shadowing and clinical hours: Many students noted that the MAPP did not provide opportunities for clinical shadowing or clinical hours. They emphasized the difficulty of getting clinical hours, especially during the COVID-19 pandemic.

Theme 2: Student community-building activities. Students noted that their community was a significant benefit of MAPP, but opportunities to get together were insufficient. They recognized the need for virtual events but felt they were disconnected and did not facilitate "peer-to-peer" community- building.

DISCUSSION

This study is one of the first mixed-methods assessments of a medical school preparatory program targeting undergraduate students from underrepresented backgrounds. It elucidates how these programs support students and any gaps in their approach. We found that students entering the program had little knowledge about, or exposure to, medical school admissions goals or procedures. Using social cognitive career theory, we found that program participants improved across all three domains: specifically, self-efficacy, outcome expectations, and personal goals. Students attested increased confidence, excitement, and knowledge, which we attribute to the professional MCAT preparation materials, workshops, and near-peer mentorship MAPP provided. We also found that the cohort's interactions gave them a sense of community and belonging, which encouraged them to apply to medical school, despite the system's lack of support for diversity.

A unique component of our evaluation method enabled us to identify critical areas for improvement and areas that most benefit students. Programs should not aim to "create doctors from diverse backgrounds"; they should promote student success, regardless of career path, which could deviate from medicine. The information and tools MAPP provides apply to many other professions or further education in fields not related to medicine. Feeling more confident, identifying community, and encouraging others within that community to succeed are crucial for the long-term success of underrepresented students in any career field.

We also show that MAPP can improve the perceived knowledge and support that underrepresented students need to feel they belong in the medical education system. Students noted that workshops showed them a review process beyond "cookie-cutter" or "box-checking", which empowered them to discuss their backgrounds, hardships, and obstacles frankly, rather than conform to standard application approaches. They learn to highlight their singular personalities, backgrounds, and experiences as assets to their medical school and future careers as physicians.

While not initially apparent, students stressed the importance of the peer community MAPP developed. Many noted a critical intangible: identifying with peers from similar backgrounds and experiencing similar discouragement and worries in applying to medical school. It gave them hope and dispelled their sense of isolation. After the program, many still work together or check in with one another about their progress. This social support cannot be generated by written materials or prerecorded lectures, and it will serve them far beyond the program. We believe that the early support of a community, carried forward during medical school and into the career, is essential to reduce dropout, encourage specialty training, and lower risk of imposter syndrome.

Several areas for improvement were identified. Students noted that COVID-19 pandemic precautions that required virtual interaction reduced their ability to create community. However, despite the virtual delivery of the MAPP studied, students still established camaraderie. We believe that adding in-person events with dedicated community-building opportunities would promote and solidify connections to foster unique and essential ties. At the same time, the convenience and atemporality of virtual interactions could provide more access to near-peer mentors of similar backgrounds and improve outcomes and external validity at other institutions.

Another area of improvement students suggested was mental health support. They noted that the medical school application process is complicated and fraught with setbacks, judgments, and harsh criticism. The current program structure focuses on providing objective, application-relevant information. It might be improved by adding sessions on achieving a growth-based mindset, incorporating failures, or preparing for extensive external evaluation.

This study had some limitations. We interviewed students in a single program at an academic medical center. Broader implementation should be adjusted to the specific demographics and cultural differences of the local community. Since participation in the interviews was completely voluntary, it may have introduced a bias by engaging students who appreciated the program more than others. Nonetheless, we interviewed over 75% of total program participants.

Similarly, a member of the OHEDI team interviewed students, which may have introduced bias. However, student comfort with the interviewer was an advantage for more open communication about program successes and failures. Furthermore, students were removed from the MAPP setting, and the interviewer had no influence on future medical school success.

Future research will explore implementation of the suggestions noted above. Specifically, we will incorporate community-building events and a clinical shadowing program to engage and enable underrepresented students to apply to medical school. A longitudinal study will focus on quantifying student success after MAPP, including medical school acceptance rates and long-term professional success.

CONCLUSIONS

Our study shows how a small program with minimal operational overhead can successfully support premedical students of diverse backgrounds in completing a medical school application. We show that MAPP participation increased their knowledge and self-esteem and provided the support they needed to feel that they belong in the medical education system. Many noted a critical intangible benefit: MAPP enabled them to form a community with peers of similar backgrounds, which gave them hope, confidence, and support. Future work will target improving community-building activities and expanding the program to more students.

REFERENCES

Agency for Health Research and Quality (AHRQ). (2017). *2017 National healthcare quality and disparities report* (pp. 1–20). Rockville, MD: AHRQ. https://www.ncbi.nlm.nih.gov/books/NBK579743/

Aibana, O., Swails, J. L., Flores, R. J., & Love, L. T. (2019). Bridging the gap: Holistic review to increase diversity in graduate medical education. *Academic Medicine: Journal of the Association of American Medical Colleges*, 94(8), 1137–1141. https://doi.org/10.1097/ACM.0000000000002779

Alsan, M., Garrick, O., & Graziani, G. (2019). Does diversity matter for health? Experimental evidence from Oakland. *American Economic Review, 109*(12), 4071–4111. https://doi.org /10.1257/aer.20181446

Association of American Medical Colleges (AAMC). (2019). *Diversity in medicine: Facts and figures 2019* (pp. 1–20). https://www.aamc.org/media/38266/download

——. (2020). *Addressing and eliminating racism at the AAMC and beyond.* https://www.aamc.org /addressing-and-eliminating-racism-aamc-and-beyond

——. (2022). *Holistic review.* https://www.aamc.org/services/member-capacity-building /holistic-review

Campbell, K. M., Rodriguez, J. E., & Berne-Anderson, T. (2014). From underrepresented minority high school student to medical school faculty member: How an outreach program changed my life. *Journal of Health Care for the Poor and Underserved, 25*(3), 972–975. https://doi.org/10.1353/hpu.2014.0137

Campbell, K. M., Bright, C. M., Corral, I., Tumin, D., & Linares, J. L. I. (2022). Increasing underrepresented minority students in medical school: A single-institution experience. *Journal of Racial and Ethnic Health Disparities.* https://doi.org/10.1007/s40615-022-01241-6

Cantor, J. C., Bergeisen, L., & Baker, L. C. (1998). Effect of an intensive educational program for minority college students and recent graduates on the probability of acceptance to medical school. *Journal of the American Medical Association, 280*(9), 772–776. https://doi .org/10.1001/jama.280.9.772

Clance, P. R., & Imes, S. A. (1978). The impostor phenomenon in high-achieving women: Dynamics and therapeutic intervention. *Psychotherapy: Theory, Research & Practice, 15*(3), 241–247.

Creswell, J. W., & Creswell, J. D. (2017). *Research design: Qualitative, quantitative, and mixed methods approaches.* Sage publications.

Grbic, D., Jones, D. J., & Case, S. T. (2015). The role of socioeconomic status in medical school admissions: Validation of a socioeconomic indicator for use in medical school admissions. *Academic Medicine, 90*(7), 953–960. https://doi.org/10.1097/ACM.0000000000000653

Keith, L., & Hollar, D. (2012). A social and academic enrichment program promotes medi-cal school matriculation and graduation for disadvantaged students. *Education for Health: Change in Learning and Practice, 25*(1), 55–63. https://doi.org/10.4103/1357-6283.99208

Lent, R. W., Brown, S. D., & Hackett, G. (2002). Social cognitive career theory. *Career Choice and Development, 4*(1), 255–311.

Musick, D. W., & Ray, R. H. (2015). Preparation for medical school via an intensive summer program for future doctors: A pilot study of student confidence and reasoning skills. *Journal of Education and Training Studies, 4*(2), 169–176. https://doi.org/10.11114/jets.v4i2.1157

Nouri, Z., Dill, M. J., Conrad, S. S., Moreland, C. J., & Meeks, L. M. (2021). Estimated prevalence of US physicians with disabilities. *JAMA Network Open, 4*(3), e211254–e211254. https://doi.org/10.1001/jamanetworkopen.2021.1254

Silver, J. K., Bean, A. C., Slocum, C., Poorman, J. A., Tenforde, A., Blauwet, C. A., Kirch, R. A., Parekh, R., Amonoo, H. L., Zafonte, R., & Osterbur, D. (2019). Physician workforce disparities and patient care: A narrative review. *Health Equity, 3*(1), 360–377. https://doi.org/10.1089/heq.2019.0040

Smedley, B. D., Stith, A. Y., & Nelson, A. R. (Eds.). (2003). *Unequal Treatment.* Institute of Medicine Committee on Understanding and Eliminating Racial and Ethnic Disparities in Health Care. https://doi.org/10.17226/12875

Takeshita, J., Wang, S., Loren, A. W., Mitra, N., Shults, J., Shin, D. B., & Sawinski, D. L. (2020). Association of racial/ethnic and gender concordance between patients and physicians with patient experience ratings. *JAMA Network Open, 3*(11), e2024583–e2024583. https://doi.org/10.1001/jamanetworkopen.2020.24583

Talamantes, E., Henderson, M. C., Fancher, T. L., & Mullan, F. (2019). Closing the gap— Making medical school admissions more equitable. *New England Journal of Medicine, 380*(9), 803–805. https://doi.org/10.1056/NEJMp1808582

United States Census Bureau (2020). *United States Census* (pp. 1–20). https://www.census.gov/programs-surveys/decennial-census/decade/2020/2020-census-main.html

Wrensford, G. E., Stewart, K.-A., & Hurley, M. M. (2019). A health professions pipeline for underrepresented students: Middle and high school initiatives. *Journal of Racial and Ethnic Health Disparities, 6*(1), 207–213. https://doi.org/10.1007/s40615-018-0515-9

Youngclaus, J., & Roskovensky, L. (2018). An updated look at the economic diversity of US medical students. *AAMC Analysis in Brief, 18*(5), 1–3.

Survey Questions

Please complete the survey below.

Thank you!

First Name	_____
Last name	_____
What is your date of birth?	_____
Which of the following best describes you?	☐ White or Caucasian ☐ Asian ☐ Native Hawaiian or Pacific Islander ☐ Black or African American ☐ Hispanic or Latinx ☐ American Indian or Alaskan Native ☐ Other
How would you describe your gender?	☐ Male ☐ Female ☐ Trans-gender ☐ Non-binary ☐ Prefer not to say ☐ Other
What year did you graduate High School?	_____
What year did you or are you planning to graduate college?	_____
What is your current college GPA?	_____
What is your intended major?	_____
How many people in your immediate family attended college?	_____
What preparation have you done for medical school prior to entering the MAPP program specifically with:	☐ MCAT prep ☐ Physician Shadowing ☐ Research ☐ Volunteer work ☐ Leadership ☐ No prior experience
What did you know about the medical school application process prior to the MAPP program?	_____
Had you participated in any medical school admissions courses or programs prior to the MAPP program?	○ Yes ○ No

If yes, how many programs and when?

_____

If no, which factors were barriers to participating in
other programs?

_____

Are you planning on participating in any other medical
application preparatory programs?

○ Yes
○ No

If yes, which ones?

_____

Current State of Combined Baccalaureate-MD Programs: A Scoping Review

Wiktoria Gocal, MD[1]; Kelly Underman, PhD[2]

Author Affiliations: [1]Department of Otorhinolaryngology, University of Maryland Medical Center, Baltimore, Maryland; [2]Department of Sociology, Drexel University, Philadelphia, Pennsylvania

Corresponding Author: Kelly Underman, Department of Sociology, Drexel University, 3201 Arch St. Suite 240, Philadelphia, PA, 19104 (*Kelly.underman@drexel.edu*)

ABSTRACT

Combined baccalaureate-Doctor of Medicine (MD) programs were developed to address the need for more—and more diverse—physicians. The authors searched three databases for articles on the subject published in the last 23 years. A total of 4,045 citations were screened, and 21 full-text articles included. Most articles (11/21, 52.4%) were published between 2000–2009, and 4/21 (19%) originated from the same program. Key themes included comparison to traditional programs; how they address societal needs; and their enhanced curricula. These programs offer solutions to current healthcare challenges, including workforce burnout and the need for diversity, equity, and inclusion in medical schools. More research on program support structures, outcomes, and curricular innovation will aid medical educators in developing and improving these programs.

Keywords: ▪ Accelerated Programs ▪ BS+MD Programs ▪ Medical Education ▪ Combined degree programs ▪ Admissions

INTRODUCTION

In the United States, combined baccalaureate-Doctor of Medicine (MD) programs offer conditionally guaranteed medical school admission to baccalaureate applicants. They were created in

J Best Pract Health Prof Divers, (Spring, 2024), 17(1), 18–33.
ISBN 2745-2843 © Winston-Salem State University

the early 1960s in response to a declining applicant pool and aim to produce more physicians in less time and to attract outstanding students, especially to primary care practices targeting medically underserved areas (Eaglen et al., 2012). While no central database encompasses all programs, an estimated 44 medical schools currently offer them (Association of American Medical Colleges [AAMC], n.d.). Program duration varies from 7–8 years, and those that shorten the baccalaureate portion are considered "accelerated".

Despite one recent review of program criteria, systematic examinations are few (Eaglen et al., 2012). This paper presents data from a scoping review of the last 23 years of research on combined baccalaureate-MD programs in the United States. It assesses findings on their strengths and weaknesses and their role in developing the future physician workforce. Given the healthcare crisis associated with the Great Recession (Margerison-Zilko, Goldman-Mellor, Falconi, & Downing, 2016) and COVID-19, when in only one month, 1.4 million healthcare jobs were lost (Teasdale, & Schulman, 2020), new educational approaches are needed to achieve an adequate primary care physician workforce, particularly to remediate disparities (Wilensky, 2022).

METHODS

Rationale

To ensure reliability and easy replication, our scoping review followed the methodological framework proposed by Arksey and O'Malley (2005) and enhanced by Levac and colleagues (Tricco et al., 2018). Findings are reported in accordance with the Preferred Reporting Items for Systematic Reviews and Meta-Analyses extension for Scoping Reviews (PRISMA-ScR) (Tricco et al., 2018).

Our search was conducted on January 12, 2023. Keywords synonymous with combined baccalaureate-MD programs were entered into the 3 electronic databases thought to be most relevant to the topic: PubMed, Web of Science (Core Collection), and ProQuest Central. We limited the scope to English-language publications dating from January 1, 2000, as significant changes in higher education occurred during this time (Hainline et al, 2010). Appendix A shows the full version of the search strategy, including keywords.

We imported and managed all citations using Rayyan online software (Ouzzani et al., 2016). The reviewer screened all results two separate times with input from the author. After removing duplicates, we screened all titles and abstracts. We then screened the full-text articles against predetermined inclusion and exclusion criteria. Inclusion mandated peer-review and publication on or after January 1, 2000. Non-US programs, accelerated nursing programs, early-assurance programs, dental school literature, and programs with a shortened MD educational portion were excluded. The resulting sample comprised 21 articles.

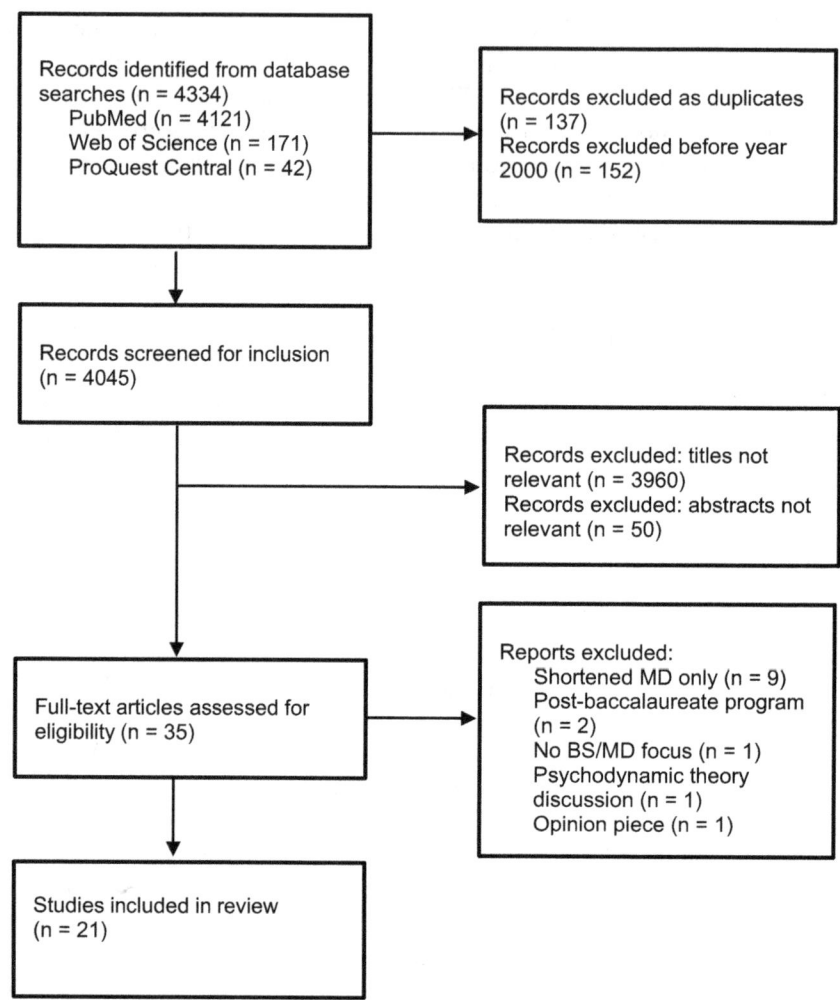

Figure 1: Excluded and included studies.

Table 1: Publication Characteristics

Publication Characteristic	No. (%) of studies (N = 21)
Publication date range	
2000–2009	11 (52.4)
2010–2019	6 (28.6)
2020–2023	4 (19.0)
Institution of origin	
University of Missouri-Kansas City School of Medicine	4 (19.0)
Warren Alpert Medical School of Brown University	3 (14.3)
City University of New York Medical School/Sophie Davis School of Biomedical Education	2 (9.5)
University of New Mexico School of Medicine	2 (9.5)
Baylor College of Medicine and the University of Texas-Pan American	2 (9.5)
University of Texas Health Science Center at San Antonio	1 (4.8)
Northwestern University Feinberg School of Medicine	1 (4.8)
Jefferson Medical College and the Pennsylvania State University	1 (4.8)

Using a descriptive-analytic model (Arksey & O'Malley, 2005), the investigator, with input from the senior author, synthesized and collated the data. Quantitative analysis focused on publication characteristics, including author, year, title, and institution of origin. For qualitative analysis, purpose/objective, methods, results/conclusions, and themes were recorded. All data were collected and organized using Microsoft Excel software. The authors then discussed the theme summaries for each study and grouped them into three distinct categories: (a) comparison to traditional programs and how they addressed (b) societal needs and (c) curriculum enhancement. Institutional Board Review approval was not required.

RESULTS

Study Characteristics. The search identified 4,045 unique titles, and 21 full-text articles were included in the final analysis. Most were published between 2000–2009 (n = 11, 52.4%), and four (19%) originated from the same program at the University of Missouri-Kansas City School of

Table 2: Publication Objectives

Author	Year	Objective
Arnold et al.	2002	UMKC School of Medicine introduced an innovative approach to geriatric education that seeks to challenge stereotypes about aging and to help students view it as a multidimensional process, learn from factors in healthy aging, and explore medical conditions of older patients.
Ballejos et al.	2019	To evaluate whether the University of New Mexico (UNM) combined baccalaureate/Medical Degree (BA/MD) program increases the likelihood that students match into family medicine residencies
Borges et al.	2007	To determine whether differences between the traditional and accelerated route groups affected career development and readiness to cope with tasks encountered in their career
Cosgrove et al.	2007	To increase recruitment and long-term retention of physicians for rural practice through a partnership between UNM SOM and College of Arts & Sciences
Drees et al.	2007	To catalog the results of a 6-year, integrated BA/MD program designed to address key educational issues inherent in traditional models and represent a community-based medical school
Eaglen et al.	2012	To describe the number, geographic distribution, institutional affiliations, missions and goals, curricula, admission and retention requirements, duration, and size of current programs
George et al.	2016	To determine any association between highly distinct premedical curricular and admission requirements and medical school performance and residency placement in two admission routes at the Warren Alpert Medical School of Brown University
Gonnella et al.	2021	To assess educational and professional outcomes of an accelerated combined BS/MD program using data collected from 1968–2018
Graves et al.	2002	To discuss implementation of a spirituality curriculum at UMKC in the 6-year combined BA-MD program; more specifically, to (a) expand students' conceptualization of the patient as a person with spiritual beliefs and needs;(b) develop an understanding of how patients' spiritual belief systems affect their health; (c) recognize how students' spiritual beliefs affect their practice of medicine;(d) highlight the value of the chaplain as a member of the healthcare team
Green et al.	2016	To compare educational outcomes of an accelerated combined baccalaureate/MD program and the traditional pathway over a 15-year period

Hagiwara et al.	2020	To identify the knowledge, skills, and any attitude changes among first-year college students in an accelerated BA/MD program after participation in an early-exposure geriatrics curriculum
Jones et al.	2000	To account for age and premedical education in determining whether male and female medical school graduates differ significantly in opinions of their medical school preparation, professional activities, and personal qualities and values
Lin et al.	2021	To examine perceptions of research and research-oriented careers among BA/MD students at Brown University
McBeth et al.	2000	To combine a freshman orientation course with academic advising as part of the combined BS-MD program at CUNY Medical School/Sophie Davis School of Biomedical Education
Merritt et al.	2021	To determine the demographics of combined program graduates and to compare their intention to practice in primary care and to work with medically underserved communities to the intentions of traditional MD program graduates
Roman	2004	To describe the Sophie Davis School of Biomedical Education 7-year, joint BS/MD program and its efforts to expand access to medical education for talented inner-city youths, including minorities and those with limited financial resources
Sirridge et al.	2003	To offer humanities courses throughout the 6-year, combined BA/MD program, hypothesizing that reading literature & writing stories helps medical students better read patient experiences
Smith	2004	To describe the meta-curricular decisions made by Brown University regarding the 8-year, combined baccalaureate-MD Program in Liberal Medical Education (PLME)
Thomson et al.	2003	To describe the development and outcomes of the Baylor College of Medicine and University of Texas-Pan American Premedical Honors College (PHC), an 8-year, BS-MD program intended to increase the number of physicians addressing the healthcare needs of underserved populations in Texas
Thomson et al.	2010	To describe the 15-year outcomes of a pipeline program to increase access to medical education for students from South Texas (a predominantly Latinx, medically underserved region), offered through Baylor College of Medicine and University of Texas-Pan American
Tran et al.	2018	To review the educational and professional development benefits of BA/MD college research, the lack of evidence-based strategies to guide program innovation, and lessons from non-US medical school research enrichment efforts and teaching models

Table 3: Publication Themes

Thematic Breakdown	No. (%) of studies (N = 21)
Comparison to traditional programs (outcome)	5 (23.8)
Ballejos et al. (family medicine residency placement)	
Borges et al. (career maturity)	
George et al. (academic performance, residency placement)	
Gonnella et al. (educational and professional outcomes)	
Green et al. (educational outcomes)	
Addressing Societal Needs	7 (33.3)
Cosgrove et al. (retention of physicians in rural New Mexico)	
Drees et al. (train more physicians in Missouri)	
Jones et al. (male vs female preparation, professional activities, qualities/values)	
Merritt et al. (intention to practice in primary care, work with medically underserved)	
Roman (increase access to medical education in New York City)	
Thomson et al., 2003, 2010 (increase access to medical education in South Texas)	
Curriculum Enhancement (intervention)	8 (38.0)
Arnold et al. (geriatrics course)	
Graves et al. (spirituality course)	
Hagiwara (geriatrics course)	
Lin et al. (research)	
McBeth et al. (academic advising)	
Sirridge et al. (medical humanities course)	
Smith (meta-curriculum)	
Tran (research engagement)	
Review of Combined Programs in United States	1 (4.8)
Eaglen et al.	

Medicine. One article was a review of US combined programs and therefore did not fit into any of the theme categories (Eaglen et al., 2012).

Theme 1 – Comparison to Traditional Programs

The first major theme identified in 5 of the 21 (23.8%) articles focused on comparing academic performance, career maturity, and professional outcomes, such as residency placement, between combined and traditional programs. Some articles compared student demographics. Ballejos et al. (2019) showed that participation in the University of New Mexico's combined baccalaureate/MD program significantly predicted matching into a family medicine residency. While the authors controlled for demographic factors that could influence specialty choice, a secondary analysis suggested combined program students had lower MCAT scores, higher overall and science GPAs, lower socioeconomic status, and were younger and more likely to come from underrepresented or rural backgrounds than all other students.

Although demographic information was not available for the population studied by Borges et al., traditional program students appeared to have greater career maturity than did combined program students. The former were thought to have already coped with the tasks of career crystallization and specification; that is, they were clearer about their preference for a specific medical career and had developed their vocational identity.

George et al. (2016) compared demographic information, academic performance, and residency placement between students pursuing a traditional premedical route and those in a combined program at the Brown University Warren Alpert Medical School. The combined program group was significantly more racially/ethnically diverse; less likely to major in a science discipline; and had completed significantly fewer premedical biology courses. Traditional students outperformed them on preclinical, shelf, and Step 1 and Step 2 exams; received more honors grades in core clerkships; and were more likely to be inducted into the Alpha Omega Alpha (AOA) honor society. No statistically significant difference was found in the competitiveness of residency programs either group matched into.

Comparing students in the combined Pennsylvania State University and Jefferson Medical College program to students in traditional programs, Gonnella et al. (2021) considered student demographics, academic progress and performance on medical licensing exams, satisfaction with medical school, educational debt, and professional outcomes, such as specialty choice, competence ratings by residency program directors, board certification rates, and faculty appointments. Combined program students were significantly younger. Substantially fewer were Caucasian and more Asian. They were less satisfied with the first three years of medical school, had lower average ratings in the area of professional attitudes, and had accrued significantly less debt. No differences were found in licensing examination performance, academic progress, specialty choice, board certification, faculty appointments, or residency program directors' ratings in six postgraduate competency areas.

The Northwestern University Feinberg School of Medicine compared the demographics of combined and traditional cohorts, focusing on academic performance and outcomes as measured by American Osteopathic Association (AOA) selection, medical licensing exams, and specialty match results (Green et al., 2016). Combined program students were younger and less likely to belong to a racial or ethnic group underrepresented in medicine. More were Asian/Pacific Islander, and fewer were White. They were significantly more likely to enter Internal Medicine and less likely to choose Emergency Medicine or Obstetrics-Gynecology. Their academic performance was comparable, and no significant differences in AOA selection or medical licensing exam performance emerged.

Theme 2 – Addressing Societal Needs

The key theme of addressing societal needs was identified in 7 (33.3%) results since many combined programs are created to expand access to medical education and medical care for underserved populations. Many combined programs strive to be community-based with the dual goal of increasing recruitment and long-term retention in specific geographic areas. Cosgrove et al. (2007) described the UNM combined program's efforts to recruit and provide students from rural and underrepresented minority populations with an academically unique and financially enhanced curriculum in hopes of increasing physician retention to improve the state's health. Similarly, Drees et al. (2007) discuss the development and implementation of the UMKC School of Medicine combined program; an estimated 45% of graduates remained in Missouri and adjacent counties in Kansas and Illinois.

The Sophie Davis School of Biomedical Education in New York City and the Premedical Honors College program in South Texas both identify the need to expand access to medical education (Roman, 2004). They focused admissions on inner-city youth who might have experienced educational disadvantage and emphasized primary care; 83% of graduates pursued primary care, and less than 1% did not earn the MD. In particular, the unique recruitment, admission, and curricular strategies of the Premedical Honors College increased (a) access to medical education for students from underrepresented and disadvantaged backgrounds; (b) retention of physicians in South Texas; and (c) overall diversity and cultural awareness and competence at Baylor College of Medicine (Thomson et al., 2003).

Identifying the need to expand medical care, Merritt et al. (2021) analyzed combined programs in terms of students' intention to practice in primary care and with the medically underserved. They found that combined program students were more likely to be relatively younger and female and less likely to identify as members of an underrepresented group. Compared to traditional program students, they were significantly more likely to intend to pursue primary care but no more likely to intend to care for the medically underserved or to practice in underserved areas. Note that the factors identified as significant predictors of the intent to work with the medically underserved included female sex, underrepresented status, and having debt.

Although somewhat outdated, a publication by Jones et al. (2000) indicates that women in combined programs are significantly more likely to practice in socioeconomically deprived areas and to treat higher percentages of low-income patients.

Theme 3 – Curriculum Enhancement

Combined programs' curriculum enhancement was a theme identified in 8 (38%) articles. Two discussed successful implementation of geriatrics courses for combined program students at two different institutions (Hagiwara et al., 2020; Jones et al., 2000). Both show improvements in student knowledge, skills, and attitudes toward older adults. The UMKC School of Medicine program wanted to challenge stereotypes about aging, teaching students to view it as multidimensional and to understand factors of healthy aging as well as medical conditions of older patients. Preclinical medical students were paired with an older adult living independently. Over 2 years, they completed projects together and engaged in conversations, and the students recorded their reflections in a journal (Arnold et al., 2002).

The geriatrics curriculum at the University of Texas Health Science Center at San Antonio aimed to identify changes in first-year college students' knowledge, skills, and attitudes toward the elderly following course participation. Before and after completing 15 interactive classes, students took a knowledge test, an attitude survey, and an objective structured clinical exam (OSCE) focusing on issues pertinent to geriatric patients.

The UMKC School of Medicine also introduced a course on spirituality and courses in the medical humanities (Graves et al., 2002; Sirridge & Welch, 2003). As part of the spirituality course, students participated in lectures, small-group activities, and an on-call experience with a hospital chaplain. At its conclusion, they were required to write reflective essays. Course participation was found to improve their understanding of the value of spirituality in healing and their intention to draw on chaplains in their future practice.

Sirridge & Welch found that various medical humanities courses offered throughout the curriculum improved students' understanding of what it means to be a good doctor, the role of human relationships in medicine, and the multidimensional nature of the healing process.

Investigators also considered research as an important curriculum enhancement strategy. Lin et al. (2021) examined perceptions of research among students in the combined program at Brown University. Overall, they viewed research and research-oriented careers positively and emphasized the importance of faculty mentorship. The most commonly identified barriers to research included lack of time, interest, or experience as well as COVID-19 isolation requirements and remote studying.

Tran et al. (2018) identified only four combined programs in the United States that required research participation and explored teaching models to boost engagement. Some effective strategies included structured research-project teamwork in the classroom, structured research experiences with faculty mentors, and clinician-researcher, skills-based workshops.

CUNY Medical School/Sophie Davis School of Biomedical Education included academic advising as part of the combined program (McBeth et al., 2000). The intervention consisted of a weekly first-year course that covered academic and societal survival skills. Results showed greater student satisfaction and improved academic performance.

Last, Smith (2004) discussed the "meta-curriculum" implemented in the Brown University combined program. It focuses on communication skills, lifelong learning, professional development, personal growth, and the social contexts of healthcare.

DISCUSSION

This scoping review's analysis of the 21 articles that met inclusion criteria educed three themes: how combined programs compare to traditional programs; how they address societal needs; and what curriculum enhancements they deploy. Overall, it demonstrates a small but strong body of empirical scholarship with important implications for combined program development and future research.

The use of such programs to enhance representation in medical education appears to depend upon the specific program. No overall patterns were identified; some programs demonstrate increased diversity; others, less than in traditional cohorts. More research is needed to define the program features that broaden participation, such as financial incentives, given that concerns about debt have been shown to restrict participation in medical education (Grace, 2017).

Combined programs seem to address society's need for primary care in medically underserved areas. Most studies on this topic demonstrate that students in combined programs are more likely to be interested in primary care or internal medicine and in working with medically underserved populations than their counterparts in traditional programs, especially when universities are able to attract and retain underrepresented students. Longitudinal research is needed to define combined program students' career pathways and contributions in areas of societal need.

Implications

This scoping review demonstrates more curricular flexibility in combined programs. Enhancements, such as content on spirituality and social determinants of health, enlarge student discernment beyond GPA and MCAT requirements. Efforts to increase programming on the social sciences and humanities, narrative medicine or the arts, and the social determinants of health or structural competency (Metzl & Hansen, 2014), may be more successful (Olsen, 2016; Olsen & Gebremariam, 2022). Premedical students are known to experience high levels of stress and competitiveness, and as more combined programs become MCAT-optional, research is needed to determine whether this strategy helps to reduce burnout (Grace, 2018). Findings are especially important given the pressing crisis of physician suicide, physicians leaving the profession, and increased demands for culturally or structurally competent and identity-concordat care (Margerison-Zilko et al., 2017; Metzl & Hansen, 2014; Street et al., 2008).

Limitations

Among the limitations of our assessment, the quality and extent of metrics the studies considered were heterogenous. In addition, most articles (52.4%) were published prior to 2009 and examined only a few institutions. The lack of a central database to track programs is a problem for any attempt to broadly analyze their effectiveness. The authors recommend the AAMC invest more resources in a systematic collection of data.

CONCLUSIONS

Initially established in the 1960s to meet pressing medical need in underserved areas and primary care and to enhance diversity in medical schools, combined baccalaureate-MD programs offer promise for similar challenges today. Can they remediate shortages due to COVID-19 burnouts and resignations? Can they help to increase diversity, equity, and inclusion in medical schools? More detailed research on program support structures, outcomes, and curricular innovation will assist medical educators in developing and improving programs to address these urgent problems.

REFERENCES

Arksey, H., & O'Malley, L. (2005). Scoping studies: Towards a methodological framework. *International Journal of Social Research Methodology, 8*(1), 19–32. https://doi.org/10.1080/1364557032000119616

Arnold, L., Shue, C. K., & Jones, D. (2002). Implementation of geriatric education into the +first and second years of a baccalaureate-MD degree program. *Academic Medicine, 77*(9), 933–934. https://doi.org/10.1097/00001888-200209000-00038

Association of American Medical Colleges (AAMC). (n.d.) Medical schools offering combined baccalaureate-MD programs, by state and program length, 2021–2022. Students & residents. https://students-residents.aamc.org/medical-school-admission-requirements/medical-schools-offering-combined-baccalaureate-md-programs-state-and-program-length-2021-2022

Ballejos, M. P., Shane, N., Romero-Leggott, V., & Sapién, R. E. (2019). Combined-baccalaureate/medical degree students match into family medicine residencies more than similar peers: A matched case-control study. *Family Medicine, 51*(10), 854–857. https://doi.org/10.22454/FamMed.2019.110812

Cosgrove, E. M., Harrison, G. L., Kalishman, S., Kersting, K. E., Romero-Leggott, V., Timm, C., Velarde, L. A., & Roth, P. B. (2007). Addressing physician shortages in New Mexico through a combined BA/MD program. *Academic Medicine, 82*(12), 1152–1157. https://doi.org/10.1097/ACM.0b013e318159cf06

Drees, B. M., Arnold, L., & Jonas, H. S. (2007). The University of Missouri-Kansas City School of Medicine: Thirty-five years of experience with a nontraditional approach to medical education. *Academic Medicine, 82*(4), 361–369. https://doi.org/10.1097/ACM.0b013e3180332f33

Dyrbye, L. N., Shanafelt, T. D., Sinsky, C. A., Cipriano, P. F., Bhatt, J., Ommaya, A., West, C. P., & Meyers, D. (2017). Burnout among health care professionals: A call to explore and address this underrecognized threat to safe, high-quality care. *NAM Perspectives, 7*(7). https://doi.org/10.31478/201707b

Eaglen, R. H., Arnold, L., Girotti, J. A., Cosgrove, E. M., Green, M. M., Kollisch, D. O., McBeth, D. L., Penn, M. A., & Tracy, S. W. (2012). The scope and variety of combined baccalaureate-MD programs in the United States. *Academic Medicine, 87*(11), 1600–1608. https://doi.org/10.1097/ACM.0b013e31826b8498

George, P., Park, Y. S., Ip, J., Gruppuso, P. A., & Adashi, E. Y. (2016). The association between premedical curricular and admission requirements and medical school performance and residency placement: A study of two admission routes. *Academic Medicine, 91*(3), 388–394. https://doi.org/10.1097/ACM.0000000000000922

Gonnella, J. S., Callahan, C. A., Erdmann, J. B., Veloski, J. J., Jafari, N., Markle, R. A., & Hojat, M. (2021). Preparing for the MD: How long, at what cost, and with what outcomes? *Academic Medicine, 96*(1), 101–107. https://doi.org/10.1097/ACM.0000000000003298

Grace, M. K. (2017). Subjective social status and premedical students' attitudes towards medical school. *Social Science & Medicine, 184*, 84–98. https://doi.org/10.1016/j.socscimed.2017.05.004

Grace, M. K. (2018). Depressive symptoms, burnout, and declining medical career interest among undergraduate pre-medical students. *International Journal of Medical Education, 9*, 302.

Graves, D. L., Shue, C. K., & Arnold, L. (2002). The role of spirituality in patient care: Incorporating spirituality training into medical school curriculum. *Academic Medicine, 77*(11), 1167. https://doi.org/10.1097/00001888-200211000-00035

Green, M. M., Welty, L., Thomas, J. X., & Curry, R. H. (2016). Academic performance of students in an accelerated baccalaureate/MD program: Implications for alternative physician education pathways. *Academic Medicine, 91*(2), 256–261. https://doi.org/10.1097/ACM.0000000000000804

Hagiwara, Y., Pagan-Ferrer, J., & Sanchez-Reilly, S. (2020). Impact of an early-exposure geriatrics curriculum in an accelerated baccalaureate-MD program. *Gerontology & Geriatrics Education, 41*(4), 508–513. https://doi.org/10.1080/02701960.2018.1464919

Hainline, L., Gaines, M., Long Feather, C., Padilla, E., & Terry, E. (2010). Changing students, faculty, and institutions in the twenty-first century. *Peer Review, 12(3),* 7–11.

Jones, B. J., Arnold, L., Xu, G., & Epstein, L. C. (2000). Differences in the preparation and practice of male and female physicians from combined baccalaureate-MD degree programs. *Journal of the American Medical Women's Association (1972), 55*(1), 29–31.

Lin, J. C., Ip, J. Y., Clark, M. A., & Greenberg, P. B. (2021). College-level baccalaureate-MD student perceptions of research and research-oriented careers. *Rhode Island Medical Journal (2013), 104*(7), 55–58.

Margerison-Zilko, C., Goldman-Mellor, S., Falconi, A., & Downing, J. (2016). Health impacts of the great recession: A critical review. *Current Epidemiology Reports, 3*(1): 81–91. doi: 10.1007/s40471-016-0068-6

McBeth, D. L., Richardson, S. M., & Cregler, L. L. (2000). The advantages of combining the freshman seminar with academic advising in an integrated BS-MD program. *Academic Medicine, 75*(9), 866. https://doi.org/10.1097/00001888-200009000-00003

Merritt, R., Baird, J., & Clyne, B. (2021). Demographics and career intentions of graduates of combined baccalaureate-MD Programs, 2010–2017: An analysis of AAMC graduation questionnaire data. *Academic Medicine, 96*(1), 108–112. https://doi.org/10.1097/ACM.0000000000003576

Metzl, J. M., & Hansen, H. (2014). Structural competency: Theorizing a new medical engagement with stigma and inequality. *Social Science & Medicine, 103,* 126–133. https://doi.org/10.1016/j.socscimed.2013.06.032

Olsen, L. D. (2016). "It's on the MCAT for a reason": Premedical students and the perceived utility of sociology. *Teaching Sociology, 44*(2), 72–83.

Olsen, L. D., & Gebremariam, H. (2022). Disciplining empathy: Differences in empathy with US medical students by college major. *Health, 26*(4), 475–494.

Ouzzani, M., Hammady, H., Federowicz, Z., & Elmagarmid, A. (2016). Rayyan—A web and mobile app for systematic reviews (5:210) [Computer software]. doi: 10.1186/s13643-016-0384-4.

Roman, S. A. (2004). Addressing the urban pipeline challenge for the physician workforce: The Sophie Davis model. *Academic Medicine, 79*(12), 1175–1183. https://doi.org/10.1097/00001888-200412000-00010

Sirridge, M., & Welch, K. (2003). The program in medical humanities at the University of Missouri-Kansas City School of Medicine. *Academic Medicine, 78*(10), 973–976. https://doi.org/10.1097/00001888-200310000-00006

Smith, S. R. (2004). The meta-curriculum in medical education. *Medicine and Health, Rhode Island, 87*(8), 236–239.

Street, R. L., O'Malley, K. J., Cooper, L. A., & Haidet, P. (2008). Understanding concordance in patient-physician relationships: Personal and ethnic dimensions of shared identity. *Annals of Family Medicine, 6*(3), 198–205.

Teasdale, B., & Shulman, K. A. (2020), Are U.S. hospitals still "recession-proof"? *New England Journal of Medicine, 383*(13), e82. doi: 10.1056/NEJMp2018846

Thomson, W. A., Ferry, P. G., King, J. E., Martinez-Wedig, C., & Michael, L. H. (2003). Increasing access to medical education for students from medically underserved communities: One program's success. *Academic Medicine, 78*(5), 454–459. https://doi.org/10.1097/00001888-200305000-00006

Tran, E. M., Ip, J., & Greenberg, P. B. (2018). Engaging college-level baccalaureate-MD students in clinical research. *Rhode Island Medical Journal (2013), 101*(7), 35–38.

Tricco, A. C., Lillie, E., Zarin, W., O'Brien, K. K., Colquhoun, H., Levac, D., et al. (2018). PRISMA extension for scoping reviews (PRISMA-ScR): Checklist and explanation. *Annals of Internal Medicine, 169*(7), 467–473. https://doi.org/10.7326/M18-0850

Wilensky, G. R. (2022). The COVID-19 pandemic and the US health care workforce. *JAMA Health Forum, 3*(1), e220001–e220001.

APPENDIX A. KEYWORDS USED IN SEARCH

PubMed

(((((((((((((((accelerated BS/MD) OR (accelerated BS/MD program)) OR (accelerated BA/MD program)) OR (accelerated baccalaureate-MD program)) OR (accelerated medical school program)) OR (accelerated three-year medical education program)) OR (BS+MD medical school program)) OR (bachelor of science-doctor of medicine program)) OR (baccalaureate doctor of medicine program)) OR (baccalaureate-MD program)) OR (combined BA/MD)) OR (combined BS/MD)) OR (combined BA/MD program)) OR (combined BS/MD program)) OR (combined baccalaureate-MD program)) OR (combined baccalaureate medical degree program)

Web of Science Core Collection

Topic option used from dropdown menu

ALL=(TS=(((((((((((((((TS=(accelerated BS/MD)) OR TS=(accelerated BS/MD program)) OR TS=(accelerated BA/MD program)) OR TS=(accelerated baccalaureate-MD program)) OR TS=(accelerated medical school program)) OR TS=(accelerated three-year medical education program)) OR TS=(BS+MD medical school program)) OR TS=(bachelor of science-doctor of medicine program)) OR TS=(baccalaureate doctor of medicine program)) OR TS=(baccalaureate-MD program)) OR TS=(combined BA/MD)) OR TS=(combined BS/MD)) OR TS=(combined BA/MD program)) OR TS=(combined BS/MD program)) OR TS=(combined baccalaureate-MD program)) OR TS=(combined baccalaureate medical degree program)))

ProQuest Central

Full text and peer reviewed filter used

"Accelerated BS/MD" OR "Accelerated BS/MD program" OR "Accelerated BA/MD program" OR "Accelerated Baccalaureate-MD program" OR "Accelerated medical school program" OR "Accelerated three-year medical education program" OR "BS+MD Medical School Program" OR "Bachelor of science-doctor of medicine program" OR "Baccalaureate doctor of medicine program" OR "Baccalaureate-MD Program" OR "Combined BA/MD" OR "Combined BS/MD" OR "Combined BA/MD program" OR "Combined BS/MD program" OR "Combined baccalaureate-MD program" OR "Combined baccalaureate medical degree program"

Assessing Concepts of Diversity, Inclusion, Cultural Competence, and Cultural Humility in Healthcare Curricula

Jennifaye V. Brown, PT, PhD, NCS[1]; Evan French, PT, DPT, MA[1]; Kathleen J. Spicer, MA[1]; Julie Suhr, PhD[1]

Author Affiliations: [1]College of Health Sciences and Professions, School of Rehabilitation and Communications Sciences, Ohio University, Athens, Ohio

Corresponding Author: Jennifaye V. Brown, College of Health Sciences and Professions, School of Rehabilitation and Communications Sciences, Ohio University, 1 Ohio University, Athens, OH 45701 (*info@jvbneuropt.com*)

ABSTRACT

Preparing the healthcare workforce to deliver person-centered care can improve health outcomes, especially for communities currently underserved. However, healthcare education program assessments may not accurately measure the knowledge, skills, and behaviors that support diversity, inclusion, cultural competence, and cultural humility. This study examined the diversity concepts in assessment items, the levels in which they were measured, and the modes used. Thirty assessments were received, and 26 analyzed. None contained the key terms *diversity, inclusion, cultural competence,* or *cultural humility,* but all contained diversity concepts, and almost half (46%) specifically referenced *social determinants of health* (SDoH). Knowledge (73%) was the level most frequently assessed followed by knowledge combined with skill (8%) or with behavior (4%); the three combined accounted for 15%. Assessment modes consisted of various formatted questions, reading assignments, group discussions, and role playing. Findings indicate a lack of explicit diversity education assessment. Furthermore, graduates are not being assessed for these proficiencies in combination, which is required for efficient and effective provider/patient interaction.

Keywords: ▪ Assessment ▪ Cultural Competence ▪ Cultural Humility ▪ Diversity ▪ Inclusion

J Best Pract Health Prof Divers, (Spring, 2024), 17(1), 34–54.
ISBN 2745-2843 © Winston-Salem State University

INTRODUCTION

Scholars forecast three trends that will impact the US healthcare workforce: 1) the majority population will be non-white by 2060; 2) one in five persons will be 65 or older by 2030, outnumbering children by 2034; and 3) the primary source of population increase will be international migration by 2030 (Vespa, Medina, & Armstrong, 2020). Ethnic and racial minorities who will comprise the future majority tend to receive inequitable healthcare services, despite advances in diagnosis and treatment (Egede, 2006). Having a diverse healthcare workforce representative of the population and knowledgeable about future cultural shifts can improve health outcomes. Since 2000, the US Department of Health and Human Services (DHHS) has charged its Secretary's Advisory Committee on Health Promotion and Disease Prevention to develop recommendations to alleviate inequities associated with access and quality of healthcare in minority communities (DHHS, 2011)

Two recommendations support the recruitment and retention of a workforce that reflects the population and is knowledgeable about diversity and inclusion concepts. The first addresses education, and the second, meeting the requirements of professional licensing boards. DHHS (2011) posits that the healthcare curriculum should emphasize person-centered care, including the cultural and linguistic competencies mandated by licensing agencies. Healthcare education programs are required to teach diversity concepts, including cultural competence and humility, equity, and inclusion, in the context of social justice (Wilbur et al., 2020) and provide support enabling students to demonstrate proficiency on licensure examinations. Passing the licensure examination assures minimal competency within the scope of practice. However, no mechanisms currently assure that practitioners have learned critical content related to diversity concepts. Assessment of these topics is the first step in preparing practitioners to provide culturally relevant, person-centered care to diverse communities.

Assessment Disconnection

A coalition of higher education institutions and private industry surveyed members (Bohanon, 2019). Results indicate that neither sector is communicating its expectations in the areas of cultural competency and inclusive leadership skills. Because they disagree on which diversity and inclusion skills are most appropriate for graduates as workplace and client demographics change, what is considered important and what is actually taught are incongruent. For example, industry respondents ranked cultural competence tenth in importance, while those in higher education ranked it third. Inclusive leadership was ranked sixth by higher education respondents and eleventh by those in industry. The top five diversity and inclusion (D&I) topics industry respondents thought students should be aware of prior to workforce entry were 1) unconscious bias; 2) collaboration across cultures; 3) microaggressions and micro-inequities; 4) organizational culture;

and 5) inclusive leadership. Higher education prioritized 1) disparities and inequities; 2) cultural competency/intelligence; 3) unconscious bias; 4) collaboration across cultures; and 5) microaggressions and micro-inequities.

Higher education assessment data could be the impetus for prioritizing D&I topics and defining course objectives and learning outcomes based on feedback from industry leaders who are assessing workplace D&I performance. Assessment data could assure a level of competency at the knowledge, skill, and behavioral levels that could resolve discrepancies between educator and employer expectations and needs.

Assessment Categories

This paper is the third of three. The second examined learning experiences in professional healthcare curricula at a midwestern university (Brown, French, Spicer & Suhr, 2021). Here, we review the types of assessments used and their correlation with student performance.

Assessment can address knowledge, skill, and/or behavior, or the affective domain. Anderson and Krathwohl (2001) identify four types of knowledge: factual, conceptual, procedural, and metacognitive. Students must know facts and be able to categorize them to conceptualize differences and similarities. Procedural knowledge entails that students know how something is done. At the metacognitive level, students should reflect and realize what they do not know in the particular context and then modify it. In healthcare, metacognitive knowledge assures self-assessment to prevent biases or skill errors. It entails planning, monitoring, and evaluating behaviors (Medina, Castleberry, & Persky, 2017).

According to Anderson and Krathwohl (2001), skill is applying what one knows in a rote manner or using decision-making to solve a problem. It refers to the execution of procedural knowledge in a fixed order that ends in a predetermined result because of a known context. In an unknown context, the student must select a procedure and make decisions to obtain a result known as implementation. Events have no fixed order, thus requiring an ongoing process of decision-making. This process is the foundation for developing the skill of clinical reasoning (Cappelletti, Engel, & Prentice, 2014; Lateel, 2018).

Behavioral assessment addresses the affective component of learning: feelings or attitudes toward the situational context. In healthcare education, students must learn how to display, acknowledge, and understand their emotions, cultural norms, values, and biases. They must learn their limitations and be able to assess their behavior critically and accept feedback (Cate & De Haes, 2000; Kadar & Thompson, 2017; Kelley, Stanke, Rabi, Kuba, & Janke, 2011; Klemenc-Ketis & Vrecko, 2014). They must understand emotions, empathy, respect, and understanding of the patient's circumstances as they relate to SDoH.

However, as healthcare is increasingly delivered by specialists, who communicate with primary providers, often through some type of technology, patients are often excluded from critical aspects of their care, such as decision-making. Therefore, when an opportunity to establish rapport and communicate with patients arises, healthcare professionals must be adept at displaying the behavioral components of interpersonal skills (Cate & De Haes, 2000).

Horvat, Horey, Romios, and Kis-Rigo (2014) found that, overall, education programs must improve the scholarship of teaching in the areas of conveying conceptual frameworks, content delivery, organizational support, and evaluation, but they provide no directive for evaluating student comprehension and display of diversity concepts in the domains of knowledge, skill, and behavior. The Inventory for Assessing the Process of Cultural Competence Among Healthcare Professionals-Student Version (IAPCC-SV©) and the Cross-Cultural Adaptability Inventory (CCAI™) have been used to assess cultural competency in occupational and physical therapy, nursing, and medical education programs (Campinha-Bacote, 2007; Kelley & Meyers, 1995). The IAPCC-SV© is a 20-item self-assessment tool indicating whether or not a healthcare student is operating at a level of cultural proficiency, competence, and awareness (Campinha-Bacote, 2007). The CCAI™ is a 50-item self-assessment tool that identifies strengths and weaknesses in the areas of emotional resilience, flexibility, openness, perceptual acuity, and personal autonomy (Kelley & Meyers, 1995). However, no evidence supports their use in outcome assessment. We have no standardized mechanism to assess the specific knowledge, skills, and behaviors mapped to the learning outcomes/objectives indicated in healthcare course syllabi.

METHODS

Rationale

This third of three studies, a descriptive analysis, determined the assessment types used to measure students' knowledge of diversity concepts and/or their application as skills and behaviors. Results provide information on student performance as indicated by the number of items answered correctly or assignments passed. They also indicate whether the assessments correspond to any components of the learning experiences identified in our second study (Brown et al., 2021b). Overall, assessment outcomes at the knowledge, skill, and/or behavioral levels show how well faculty are preparing graduates to treat diverse populations.

This retrospective qualitative process of describing data content used an exploratory framework based on original data gathered in part two of this research series (Brown et al., 2021b). Exploratory research adduces evidence as defined by the subject matter (Behrens, 1997). The subject matter levels are knowledge, skill, and behavior, and mode describes type of assessment.

Setting and Sampling Strategy

As previously reported, our three-part study did not enroll human subjects and it was approved by the university's Institutional Review Board (Brown, Spicer, & French, 2021). This third segment required the review of learning experiences previously mapped to learning outcomes/course objectives for 20 courses taught at a midwestern university's health sciences college. We requested assessment items from the 49 learning experiences that met inclusion criteria.

Data Collection

Data were collected from January 13 to June 30, 2020. We have described the analysis confirming that the learning experiences contained the keywords or related words or concepts (Brown et al., 2021b). Instructors of record (IoRs) who submitted the learning experiences were asked to email us all assessment components, including the assessment items corresponding to each; a rubric, if appropriate; and the number of students who answered the individual item correctly or scored a "C" or better on an assignment, test, quiz, and/or clinical lab practicum.

Confirmation of Validity and Reliability

We used triangulation and peer review to assure the validity of our data process and an audit trail and journaling to assure reliability. Details are presented in Brown et al. (2021a).

Data Analysis

Analysis was conducted in three phases. In phase 1, the submitted assessment item was scrutinized for evidence of the keywords (diversity, inclusion, cultural competency, and cultural humility) and related words, phrases, or concepts addressed in the corresponding learning experience and identified in the codebook established in our earlier research (Brown et al., 2021a).

In phase 2, we determined the level of the assessment (knowledge, skill, or behavior). We defined a knowledge assessment as factual, conceptual, procedural, and/or metacognitive (Anderson & Krathwohl, 2001). A skill assessment measures how well a procedure is accurately executed or implemented in response to a decision about the clinical situation. A behavioral assessment demonstrates an affective component, covering domains related to communication and consideration of patient characteristics associated with SDoH, such as economic stability, education, health and healthcare, neighborhood and built environment, and social and community context (DHHS, 2010). Provider's feelings or attitudes about the situation, the patient, and themselves are also considered.

In phase 3, we defined assessment mode as the delivery format: a written or oral examination or discussion; a video analysis of a clinical situation; and/or role-playing in a clinical situation. We also considered whether the assessment was administered to an individual or a group as an assignment or a didactic or clinical lab practical competency assessment. A didactic assessment - for example, a written multiple-choice, short-answer, or true/false examination - might require students to recall, apply, analyze, evaluate, and/or create an approach to demonstrate competence. A clinical lab practical assessment could involve proficient, hands-on engagement of the concept based on recollection, analysis, examination, evaluation, application, and/or improvisation.

The primary investigator (PI) and trained research assistants separately conducted content analysis and then compared findings. Any disagreement over mapping the assessment to a learning experience, level, or mode was resolved through further discussion. If warranted, the IoR was asked to clarify how the assessment content corresponded to the learning experience.

RESULTS

Part 1 of the study identified 79 learning outcomes/course objectives and 6 other content items in 32 eligible course syllabi that contained keywords or related words/phrases or concepts (Brown, et al., 2021a). In part 2, keywords or related words/phrases or concepts were identified in 49 learning experiences (Brown et al., 2021b) and mapped to 28 learning outcomes/course objectives and 3 other items in 20 eligible course syllabi (see Table 1). Of the 49 assessments requested, 30 (61%) were received. Four had no keywords or related words/phrases or concepts corresponding to the respective learning experiences and were deemed ineligible as indicated by the dash sign (see Table 1). None of the remaining 26 (49%) assessments contained the keywords, but all contained diversity-related concepts. We categorized 11 (46%) under the five key SDoH: economic stability, health and healthcare, neighborhood and built environment, education, and/ or social and community context (DHHS, 2010; see Table 2, column 3).

Overall, 25 (96%) of the assessments were directly mapped to learning experiences, and 23 of the learning experiences were mapped to the learning outcomes/course objectives across 15 eligible course syllabi as follows: Communication Sciences and Disorders (CSD) (n=1), Exercise Physiology (EXPH) (n=4), Interdisciplinary Health Studies (IHS) (n=2), Nutrition (NUTR) (n=2), and Physical Therapy (PT) (n=6).

Two assessments had two parts; one, NUTR1, was graded for a score; and NURS1 was not, but every student completed both. Three additional assessments (EXPH4, EXPH6, NURS6) awarded no score for a grade, and all students completed them (Table 3, column 6). Of these five assessments identified by completion, one was a group effort (EXPH4); two were individual (EXPH6 and NURS6); and one had both an individual and a group component (NURS1) (Table 3, column 5).

The percentage of students answering the remaining 21 assessments correctly, or scoring a "C" or better, ranged from 68.57% to 100% (Table 3, column 6). For three (PT2:General, PT5:Neurology, and PT7:Orthopedic), the IoR did not report individual assessment item data but rather indicated the percentage of students passing the didactic examination with a score of "C" or better (Table 3, column 6). Of the 18 graded item-specific assessments, 16 measured

Table 1: Assessment Data

Course (n=20)	Eligible Syllabi: Learning Outcomes/Course Objective or Other Content Identifier	Eligible Learning Experiences	Assessment Status
CSD2: Diagnosis	1	2	1
	2	2	1
EXPH2: Section 101 Exercise Lecture	5	1	1
EXPH3: Sections 103-104 Exercise Lab	5	1	*
EXPH4: Fitness	Week 3: 9/10	2	1
EXPH5: Motor Skill	7	1	1
EXPH6: Research	3	1	1
IHS1: Prefatory	Week 6: 10/1 & 10/3	1	*
	Week 8: 10/17	2	1
	2	1	1
IHS2: Interprofessionalism	2	1	1
	4	3	*
NURS1: Introductory Reasoning	10	2	2
NURS6: Research	2	2	1
	4	2	.
NUTR1: Prefatory	9	1	*
	11	1	2
NUTR2: Professionalism	1	1	1
	4	2	1
NUTR3: Medicinal	7	1	1
	9	1	1
PT2: General	3	1	1
PT3: Business	7	1	1

PT4: Neurology	9	1	*
PT5: Neurology	3	1	1
	4	1	1
PT7: Orthopedic	5	2	-
	7	2	1
PT8: Orthopedic	4	4	1
PT9: Orthopedic	1	4	1
	9	1	1
Total	31	49	26

Note. * = No submission; - = Ineligible; CSD = Communication Sciences & Disorders; EXPH = Exercise Physiology; IHS = Interdisciplinary Health Studies; NURS = Nursing; NUTR = Nutrition; PT = Physical Therapy.

individual merit, and two, groups (NUTR3 and PT9). For NUTR3, the IoR requested that each student complete the assignment individually and as a group, submit a final document that would be graded, and each student would receive the same score (Table 3, column 5).

Of the total 26 assessments, the syllabi of 15 labeled them as assignments (two had two parts); 3, as clinical lab practical examinations; and the remaining 6, as didactic examinations (Table 3, column 5).

Knowledge, skills, and/or affective behaviors were evaluated via assignments or examination, didactic or practical. All 26 assessments contained a knowledge component of which 19 (73%) used an individual format, 13 (68%) were assignments; three (16%) multiple-choice questions; six (23%) short-answer questions; and one (5%) a true/false question. Assignments consisted of completing standardized, online multiple-choice tests; providing written short answers to questions; reading and identifying descriptors of diversity terms/concepts; and documenting a clinical case study. Knowledge was combined with skill in two (8%) of the 26 assessments and once with behavior (4%). In assessments that had a behavioral component, students interacted in group discussions (NURS1). When combined with skill, students demonstrated the proper execution or implementation of a procedure/activity (PT5 and PT8, respectively). Four (15%) of the 26 assessments addressed knowledge, skill, and behavior in group activities for a communication assignment (EXPH4), a human resources assignment (PT3), and a lab practicum and an ergonomic assignment focused on patient/provider relationships (PT9) (Table 3, columns 4 and 5).

Various modes were used. The most common were examination or assignment questions in a short-answer (23%), multiple-choice (12%), or true/false (4%) format. Discussions, either verbal

Table 2: Diversity-Related Content Connecting Assessments to Learning

Course	Assessment Number	Assessment Content	Learning Experience Content
CSD2: Diagnosis	1	Diversity concepts related to social determinants of health (SDoH): economics, health and healthcare	**Cultural** biases discussing the impact of poverty and the opioid crisis
	2	Related diversity concepts: language used at home versus among peers	Instances of **cultural**/linguistic **diversity** in practice
EXPH2: 101 Lecture	3	Related diversity concepts: age	Age, physical disability, overweight, obesity
EXPH4: Fitness	4	Related diversity concepts: teaching - verbal, visual, and kinesthetic communication styles	Communication - delivery of information specific to the individual
EXPH5: Motor Skill	5	Related diversity concepts: skill characteristics - novice to expert	Clients - high-level performers (experts)
EXPH6: Research	6	Related diversity concepts: ethical research practice - protections in human subjects research	Ethical issues in research; **culture** in communication
IHS1: Prefatory	7	Related diversity concepts: intersectionality	Intersectionality
	8	Related diversity concepts: stereotype	Stereotype
IHS2:	9	Diversity concepts related to SDoH: social and community context - advocacy	**Cultural** beliefs; **cultural** differences; healthcare inter-professionalism
NURS1: Reasoning	10 and 11	Related diversity concepts: age, social status, gender, religion, and occupation	Cross-**cultural** nursing considerations; **cultural competency**; **diverse** populations: racial, gender, social status and ethnic disparities; **culture** in various contexts; becoming a **culturally competent** nurse

NURS6: Research	12	Related diversity concepts: ethical considerations and human subjects' protections	Ethical practice, misconduct, and hospital patients
NUTR1: Prefatory	13 and 14	Diversity concepts related to SDoH: nutrition	Nutrition
NUTR2: Professionalism	15	Related diversity concepts: nutrition healthcare professionals - settings	Nutrition healthcare professionals - settings
	16	Related diversity concepts: nutrition healthcare professionals - roles	Nutrition healthcare professionals - roles; age, and medical diagnoses
NUTR3: Medicinal	17	Diversity concepts related to SDoH: nutrition healthcare, and social and community context	Religious/**cultural** aspects of diet
	18	Diversity concepts related to SDoH: nutrition, healthcare, education, and economic stability	Social and community context aligned with patient/client lifestyle
PT2: General	19	Related diversity concepts: interacting with a person who is deaf	**Cultural** knowledge: address person who is deaf by learning to work with an interpreter
PT3: Business	20	Related diversity concepts: communication skills to interview and hire qualified personnel	Develop hiring materials compliant with applicable laws
PT5: Neurology	21	Diversity concepts related to SDoH: neurologic diagnoses treatment interventions, and education - patient-centered instruction	Neurologic diagnosis and treatment interventions
	22	Diversity concepts related to SDoH: neurologic diagnoses and treatment interventions	Neurologic diagnoses and treatment interventions

(Continued)

Table 2: (*Continued*)

Course	Assessment Number	Assessment Content	Learning Experience Content
PT7: Orthopedic	23	Diversity concepts related to SDoH: orthopedic impairment and treatment interventions	Orthopedic impairment across the lifespan
PT8: Orthopedic	24	Diversity concepts related to SDoH: patient/client-centered plan of care	Person-centered care
PT9: Orthopedic	25	Diversity concepts related to SDoH: role-play patient/ client and role-play evaluating physical therapist	Orthopedic impairment and person-centered care
	26	Diversity concepts related to SDoH: low back pain and built environment - ergonomic adaptations for space	Low back pain and neighborhood and built environment

Note. The keywords diversity, inclusion, cultural competence, and/or cultural humility or variations that appear in the learning experience content are in boldface. SDoH = social determinants of health.

within a group (NURS1) or written individually and submitted to the Blackboard Learning Management System (BLMS) discussion board (IHS2), were also used. Students engaged in discussions to complete group projects (NUTR3 & PT9) and, in an assignment, to display understanding of communication styles (EXPH4). In one class, they interacted to adapt the environment based on an ergonomic case (PT9). Individually, students engaged in self-directed and organizing tasks to arrive at some result; for example, tracking their own nutritional intake over three days (NUTR1). Assessments required that students confirm their knowledge of information taught in class, looking for use of the keywords or related words or concepts in documents to be read and thereafter uploaded their written responses to BLMS (IHS1) and/or producing a document that exemplified components of a concept via clinical documentation (CSD2 and NUTR3) and patient education (NUTR3). Last, PT5, PT8, and PT9 assessed student psychomotor proficiency in playing the role of a healthcare professional in a clinical lab practical examination (Table 3, column 5).

DISCUSSION

This study was designed to identify assessments that addressed diversity concepts. Although they lacked the keywords *inclusion, cultural competency, cultural humility,* and *diversity,*

Table 3: Learning Outcomes Mapped to Assessment by Level, Mode, & Outcome

Course	Eligible Learning Outcomes/Course Objective or Other Syllabus Content Identifier	Assessment Number	Assessment Level	Assessment Mode	Assessment Outcome
CSD2: Diagnosis	1	1	K	Assignment: Write a case history using documentation standards	24/35 or 68.57% scored C or better
	2	2	K	Multiple-choice question	35/35 or 100% answered correctly
EXPH2: 101 Lecture	5	3	K	Multiple-choice question	24/24 or 100% answered correctly
EXPH4: Fitness	Week 3: 9/10	4	K, S & B	Group assignment: In-class demonstration of communication styles	29/29 or 100% completed the class activity
EXPH5: Motor Skill	7	5	K	Short-answer question	38/45 or 84.44% answered question correctly
EXPH6: Research	3	6	K	Assignment: Complete online CITI Training for Biomedical Researcher & Conflict of Interest	11/11 or 100% completed online assignment; average score 89%
IHS1: Prefatory	Week 8: 10/17	7	K	Assignment: Identify descriptors that define intersectionality	16/18 or 88.88% passed with C or better
	2	8	K	Assignment: Cite sources containing stereotypes and upload to BLMS	17/18 or 94.44% passed with B or better
IHS2: Inter-professionalism	2	9	K	Assignment: BLMS discussion board entry and written journal entry	10/12 or 83.33% passed with C or better with average 87%

(Continued)

Table 3: (*Continued*)

Course	Eligible Learning Outcomes/Course Objective or Other Syllabus Content Identifier	Assessment Number	Assessment Level	Assessment Mode	Assessment Outcome
NURS1: Introductory Reasoning	10	10	K	Assignment:	18/18 or 100% successfully completed the assignment
		11	K & B	Part 1, Individual: 6 short-answer questions pertaining to 5 scenarios Part 2, Group: discussion among students	
NURS6: Research	2	12	K	Assignment: Complete online CITI Training for Biomedical Researcher & Conflict of Interest	68/68 or 100% completed assignment & received 20 points
NUTR1: Prefatory	11	13	K	Assignment:	128/131 or 97.70% passed with a C or better
		14	K	Part 1: Final project submission Part 2: 10 Short-answer questions	
NUTR2: Professionalism	1	15	K	Assignment: 3 short-answer questions	40/44 or 90.90% passed with a C or better
	4	16	K	Assignment: 14 short-answer questions	40/44 or 90.90% passed with a C or better
NUTR3: Medicinal	7	17	K	Group assignment: ADIME documentation	24/26 or 92.30% passed with a C or better
	9	18	K	Assignment: Develop educational session/ strategy for a specific diagnosis	26/26 or 100% passed with a C or better
PT2: General	3	19	K	Multiple-choice question	46/46 or 100% passed exam with a C or better; no data for individual assessment item
PT3: Business	7	20	K, S & B	Assignment: Students perform in-person interview, then offer or deny position via phone	11/11 or 100% passed with a C or better on assignment

Course	#	Domain	Assessment	Benchmark
PT5: Neurology	3	K & S	Lab Practical Skill Execution: VOMS or BPPV assessment & treatment	16/16 or 100% passed with a C or better
	4	K	True/False question	16/16 or 100% passed exam with a C or better; no data for individual assessment item
PT7: Orthopedic	7	K	Final exam case scenario; short-answer question	43/43 or 100% passed exam with a C or better; no data for individual assessment item
PT8: Orthopedic	4	K & S	Lab practical component: document plan of care for lumbar spine	38/38 or 100% passed with a C or better
PT9: Orthopedic	1	K, S & B	Lab practical component: TMJ examination & evaluation to determine initial disposition	38/38 or 100% passed with a C or better
	9	K, S & B	In-class group assignment: three students assess and adapt ergonomics of work, home, or school environment; present adaptations and rationale	38/38 or 100% passed with a C or better

Note. CSD = Communication Sciences & Disorders; EXPH = Exercise Physiology; IHS = Interdisciplinary Health Studies; NURS = Nursing; NUTR = Nutrition; PT = Physical Therapy; K = Knowledge; S = Skill; B = Behavior (Affective Domain); CITI = Collaborative Institutional Training Initiative; BLMS = Blackboard Learning Management System; ADIME = Assessment, Diagnosis, Intervention, and Monitoring/Evaluation; VOMS = Vestibular/Ocular-Motor Screening; BPPV = Benign Paroxysnal Positional Vertigo; TMJ = Temporomandibular Joint. Adapted from Brown, Spicer, & French (2021).

results indicate that 25 (96%) mapped to relevant learning experiences. Of the 16 item-specific assessments graded individually and the two graded as a group, 15 students (94%) met the requirement of a passing grade "C" or above.

Assessments reflected three styles of learning: visual, auditory, and kinesthetic (Kharb, Samanta, Jindal, & Singh, 2013). Information recall may be assisted by the content embedded in multiple-choice answers, but a short-answer question requires students to draw, write, or type the answer, demonstrating proficiency without cues. For example, in PT7, the short-answer question required students to draw a diagram and explain the function of the labeled items. Verbal discussion can prompt recall for those with an auditory learning style. Asking questions and getting a verbal response during a clinical lab practical examination can guide the discourse. Last, performing hands-on psychomotor skills, either following rote memory or making decisions based on the situational context, exemplifies kinesthetic learning. Healthcare is a very hands-on profession, and competence in clinical skill delivery is expected as the definitive assessment format. Out of 20 eligible courses, six had a clinical lab component, and three of them used clinical practical examinations for assessment.

Diversity comprises differences in race, ethnicity, cultural norms, experience, age, language, dialect, socioeconomic status, family dynamics, educational/career aspirations, religious/political beliefs, sexual orientation, gender, physical appearance, attire, and physical ability (Bleich, MacWilliams, & Schmidt, 2015; Mazur, 2010; Smith, 2016). These assessments rarely addressed characteristics that make people or situations diverse, but rather contained the characteristic roles graduates will experience as practitioners.

Healthcare practitioners must be able to perform layered assessments and evaluate the data to justify, explain, and implement a person-centered plan of care for the best health outcomes in their respective fields. For example, in NUTR1, students completed an individual project, performing a nutrition assessment on themselves and then answering questions related to the process, the content, and the results. The process paralleled what nutritionists do with a patient: explaining the purpose, gathering and evaluating the data for content related to health status, and explaining the results. Completing short-answer questions after the assignment guided students in prioritizing and presenting information.

In physical therapy education, experiential learning relies on simulation, integrated clinical experiences (clinical rotations interspersed during didactic portions of the curriculum), service learning (voluntary opportunities to provide a service applying healthcare knowledge as a way to learn), use of community patient-resource groups, and professional practice opportunities (Smith & Crocker, 2017). None of the assessments took advantage of experiential learning in these formats but expressed components of what makes it a valuable assessment method in various ways. First, students performed healthcare practitioner tasks for assignments and second, conducted clinical lab practical examinations. The group ergonomic assignment for PT9 included playing the role of a PT redesigning the space for a patient with spinal pathology. Students were graded on their rationale for, and presentation of, the changes. Role-playing was also used to assess professional communication in PT3: students acting as managers reviewed job applications and interviewed students acting as applicants, then phoned them to tell them whether they were hired.

The clinical lab practical examination provides a supervised setting in which students can receive feedback on their role play, which can shape their future cultural competence in real-world contexts. Two courses (PT5 and PT9) used role-play in clinical lab practical examinations. The PT5 lab required students to assess and treat a vestibular pathology. In PT9, students played the role of a patient reporting an impairment or a PT taking the history, performing an exam, evaluating the results, developing a plan of care, and implementing a home exercise program. Supervision and feedback (Smith & Crocker, 2017) during a timed assessment allow students to make an error in a safe space prior to interacting with patients. By reflecting on the feedback, they can generate an approach to critique their thought processes and behaviors to improve performance. It incentivizes learning by doing. If assessment experiences enable students to recognize how diversity, inclusion, cultural competence, and cultural humility affect healthcare delivery and outcomes, then perhaps they will provide equitable care and reduce disparities.

Clear communication can reduce medical errors that compromise outcomes (Pope, Rodzen, & Spross, 2008; Risser et al., 1999). Developing the skill to transmit, justify, and explain information accurately is imperative for the patient/provider relationship and the collaboration of the healthcare team (Ruddy & Drossman, 2020). Level of trust in the provider contributes to the patient's adherence to recommendations and, thus, healthcare outcomes (Dale, Polivka, Chaudry, & Simmonds, 2010; Street, O'Malley, Cooper, & Haidet, 2008; Thornton, Powe, Roter, & Cooper, 2011). NURS1 assessed communication constructs. Each student answered questions pertaining to five scenarios in which diversity related to the person, environment, or situation played a role. They then discussed the rationale for their responses. Answers were not right or wrong, and all students received activity points for participation. The IoR reported, "This class does not have quizzes/exams. All students passed these activities. We base these activity points on participation/engagement/completion and discuss the answers. We do not grade for correctness." The emphasis was on communication, using clinical reasoning and critical thinking to answer questions based on case content and additional information found on a website. Students not only recognized diversity in terms of person, task, and context, but conducted further research to clarify and defend its meaning.

Following experiential learning activities, self-reflective writing was used to explore group dynamics among different cultural entities. In a study by Kratzke and Bertolo (2013), co-facilitators led a debriefing session after students had reflected in writing. They discussed their perceptions of cultural knowledge, cultural awareness, cultural encounters, and cross-cultural communication. In our study, the IHS2 IoR used written journal assignments and submissions to electronic discussion boards to articulate critical thinking and clinical reasoning strategies. Students reflected on the learning experience and its relationship to interprofessionalism. In another assessment assignment, IHS1 students wrote comments about the portrayal of Appalachian people in poems and what descriptors identified as stereotypes say about the region. The process of recognizing first then understanding a word's meaning in a different context develops critical thinking and reasoning.

Because practitioners must rely on accurate self-assessment throughout their careers, students must master it (Antonelli, 1997). Through self-reflection in the moment, an example of metacognition (Sullivan & Hall, 1997), students establish a process of self-assessment. It transforms them from novice to expert by improving their integrity (Driscoll, 1994; Koshy, Gundogan, Whitehurst, & Jafree, 2017). Self-assessment is a method of self-directed learning, a proactive investigation of what was done, how it was done, and whether it could be done better. By similarly being aware of and questioning the patient's verbal and physical manifestations, students develop confidence in their clinical reasoning (Lateef, 2018; Marcum 2012). However, while self-reflection improves quality of care and closes the gap between the theoretical concepts of didactic education and what actually happens in practice (Driscoll, 1994; Koshy et al., 2017), none of the three clinical lab practical examinations assessed it. Some evidence indicates that if time is of the essence, self-reflection is not seen as a priority in clinical mentoring (Kinsella, 2009). Teaching self-reflection during the didactic portion of healthcare education can enhance self-discovery and lifelong learning to improve healthcare delivery.

Limitations

Data collection was compromised by the ongoing impact of COVID-19. Despite three major recruiting efforts, limited initial enrollment of program courses resulted in only 23 assessments that could be mapped to the original learning outcomes/course objectives and syllabus content. As an exploratory study, the results cannot be applied to healthcare curricula; however, the process used to identify the keywords and related words/phrases or concepts in learning outcomes/course objectives, learning experiences, and assessments can be duplicated for comparative analysis of healthcare education programs.

Implications

Study results can be used to train healthcare faculty to teach diversity concepts prior to the licensure exam and to design assessments that assure competence upon entering the workforce. Aggregate data from licensure boards regarding content areas with the lowest passing or non-passing rate indicate which educational methods to change. This data attest the need to clarify learning outcomes/course objectives and to devise learning experiences that accommodate different learning styles. Course evaluations can substantiate best practices in teaching and assessing these concepts.

CONCLUSIONS

Professional healthcare organizations expect the workforce to reflect the population served. To that end, they expect that graduate competence in the practice of diversity concepts has been determined by objective assessment of their knowledge, skills, and behaviors. This pilot study was designed to determine whether assessments addressed diversity and found that 96% were mapped to diversity-related learning experiences; although they did not use the keywords, all contained diversity-related words/phrases, concepts, or contexts to assess knowledge, skill, and or affective behaviors demonstrating students' awareness of their role in healthcare delivery and the value of patients' perspectives. The 25 mapped assessments aligned with what was taught in the learning experience, and 23 of the learning experiences aligned with learning outcomes/ course objectives and syllabus content. Five assessments were not graded for a score but rather as completed by 100% of the students. With the exception of one assessment item in one course, all students passed the remaining 17 assessments. They were graded either as individuals (15) or as a group (2). As indicators of student performance, assessments used four modes: visual memory (multiple-choice questions, with correct answers embedded in the choices), recall (short answer to a question), and auditory stimuli (discussion groups responding to questions/commentary) for didactic examinations, or kinesthetic response (performing a psychomotor skill in a clinical lab practical examination).

This novel three-part study should be replicated on a larger scale to determine the presence of diversity related issues in the mapping of learning outcomes/course objectives of increasing complexity to learning experiences that involve knowledge, skill, and behaviors and subsequently assessed at those respective levels of increasing complexity, particularly in sequential courses. Furthermore, what is assessed as part of the program curriculum should be correlated with workforce expectations and patient outcomes.

REFERENCES

Anderson, L. W., & Krathwohl, D. R. (Eds.). (2001). *A taxonomy for learning, teaching and assessing: A Revision of Bloom's taxonomy of educational objective.* Addison Wesley Longman, Inc.

Antonelli, M. A. (1997). Accuracy of second-year medical students' self-assessment of clinical skills. *Academic Medicine, 72*(10 Suppl 1), S63–65. https://doi.org/10.1097/00001888 -199710001-00022

Behrens, J. T. (1997). Principles and procedures of exploratory data analysis. *Psychological Methods, 2*(2), 131–160. https://doi.org/10.1037/1082-989X.2.2.131

Bleich, M. R., MacWilliams, B. R., & Schmidt, B. J. (2015). Advancing diversity through inclusive excellence in nursing education. *Journal of Professional Nursing, 31*(2), 89–94. https://doi .org/10.1016/j.profnurs.2014.09.003

Bohanon, M. (2019, September). *New higher education-industry alliance will transform how we prepare students for 21ˢᵗ century careers.* Insight Into Diversity. https://www.insightintodiversity .com/new-higher-education-industry-alliance-will-transform-how-we-prepare-students-for -21st-century-careers/

Brown, J. V., Spicer, K. J., & French, E. (2021a). Exploring the inclusion of cultural competence, cultural humility, and diversity concepts as learning objectives or outcomes in healthcare curricula. *Journal of Best Practices in Health Professions Diversity, 14*(1), 63–81. https://www.jstor.org/stable/27097337

Brown, J. V., French, E., Spicer, K. J., & Suhr, J. (2021b). Teaching concepts of diversity, inclusion, cultural competence, and cultural humility through learning experiences in healthcare curricula. *Journal of Best Practices in Health Professions Diversity, 14*(2), 147–177. https://www.jstor.org/stable/27203548

Campinha-Bacote, J. (2007). *Inventory for Assessing the Process of Cultural Competence*-Student version. http://transculturalcare.net/iapcc-sv/

Cappelletti, A., Engel, J. K., & Prentice, D. (2014). Systematic review of clinical judgement and reasoning in nursing. *Journal of Nursing Education, 53*, 453–458. https://doi.org/10.3928/01484834-20140724-01

Cate, Th. J. ten, & DE HAES, J. C. J. M. (2000). Summative assessment of medical students in the affective domain. *Medical Teacher, 22*(1), 40–3. https://doi.org/10.1080/01421590078805

Dale, H., Polivka, B., Chaudry, R., & Simmonds, G. (2010). What young African American women want in a health care provider. *Qualitative Health Research, 20*(11), 1484–1490. https://doi.org/doi: 10.1177/1049732310374043

Driscoll, J. (1994). Reflective practice for practice. *Senior Nurse, 14*(1), 47–50.

Egede, L. E. (2006). Race, ethnicity, culture, and disparities in health care. *Journal of General Internal Medicine, 21*(6), 667–669. https://doi.org/10.1111/j.1525-1497.2006.0512.x

Horvat, L., Horey, D., Romios, P., & Kis-Rigo, J. (2014). Cultural competence education for health professionals. *Cochrane Database of Systematic Reviews, (5)*, CD009405. https://doi.org/10.1002/14651858.CD009405.pub2

Kadar, G. E., & Thompson, G. (2017). Assumed or assessed? The affective domain in health care education. *Journal of Nutritional Health & Food Engineering, 6*(4), 117–118. https://doi.org/10.15406/jnhfe.2017.06.00207

Kelley, C., & Meyers, J. (1995). *The Cross-Cultural Adaptability Inventory: Manual.* National Computer System, Inc.

Kelley, K. A., Stanke, L. D., Rabi, S. M., Kuba, S. E., & Janke, K. K. (2011). Cross-validation of an instrument for measuring professionalism behaviors. *American Journal of Pharmaceutical Education, 75*(9), 179. https://doi.org/10.5688/ajpe759179

Kharb, P., Samanta, P. P., Jindal, M., & Singh, V. (2013). The learning styles and the preferred teaching-learning strategies of first year medical students. *Journal of Clinical and Diagnostic Research, 7*(6), 1089–1092. https://doi.org/10.7860/JCDR/2013/5809.3090

Kinsella, E. A. (2009). Professional knowledge and the epistemology of reflective practice. *Nursing Philosophy, 11*, 3–14. https://doi.org/10.1111/j.1466-769X.2009.00428.x

Klemenc-Ketis, Z., & Vrecko, H. (2014). Development and validation of a professionalism assessment scale for medical students. *International Journal of Medical Education, 5*, 205–211. https://doi.org/10.5116/ijme.544b.7972

Koshy, K., Limb, C., Gundogan, B., Whitehurst, K., & Jafree, D. (2017). Reflective practice in health care and how to reflect effectively. *International Journal of Surgery Oncology, 2*(6), e20. https://doi.org/10.1097/IJ9.0000000000000020

Kratzke, C., & Bertolo, M. (2013). Enhancing students' cultural competence using cross-cultural experiential learning. *Journal of Cultural Diversity, 20*(3), 107–111.

Lateef, F. (2018). Clinical reasoning: The core of medical education and practice. *International Journal of Emergency Medicine, 1*(2), 1–7.

Marcum, J. A. (2012). An integrated model of clinical reasoning: Dual-process theory of cognition and metacognition. *Journal of Evaluation in Clinical Practice, 18*(5):954–961. https://doi.org/10.1111/j.1365-2753.2012.01900.x

Mazur, B. (2010). Cultural diversity in organisational theory and practice. *Journal of Intercultural Management, 2*(2), 5–15.

Medina, M. S., Castleberry, A. N., & Persky, A. M. (2017). Strategies for improving learner metacognition in health professional education. *American Journal of Pharmaceutical Education, 81*(4), Article 78. https://doi.org/10.5688/ajpe81478

Pope, B. B., Rodzen, L., & Spross, G. (2008). Raising the SBAR. How better communication improves patient outcomes. *Nursing, 38*(3), 41–43. https://doi.org/10.1097/01.nurse.0000312625.74434.e8

Risser, D. T., Rice, M. M., Salisbury, M. L., Simon, R., Jay, G. D., & Berns, S. D. (1999). The potential for improved teamwork to reduce medical errors in the emergency department. The MedTeams Research Consortium. *Annals of Emergency Medicine, 34*(3), 373–383. https://doi.org/10.1016/s0196-0644(99)70134-4

Ruddy, J., & Drossman, D. A. (2020). Improving patient-provider relationships to improve health care. *Clinical Gastroenterology and Hepatology, 18*, 1417–1426. https://doi.org/10.1016/j.cgh.2019.12.007

Smith, K. R. (2016). Teaching and learning "respect" and "acceptance" in the classroom. In M. Bart (Ed.), *Faculty focus special report: Diversity and inclusion in the college classroom* (pp. 17–19). Magna Publications.

Smith, S. N., & Crocker, A. F. (2017). Experiential learning in physical therapy education. *Advances in Medical Education and Practice, 8*, 427–433. https://doi.org/10.2147/AMEP.S140373

Street, Jr., R. L., O'Malley, K. J., Cooper, L. A., & Haidet, P. (2008). Understanding concordance in patient-physician relationships: Personal and ethnic dimensions of shared identity. *Annals of Family Medicine, 6*(3), 198–205. https://doi.org/10.1370/afm.821

Sullivan, K., & Hall, C. (1997). Introducing students to self-assessment. *Assessment & Evaluation in Higher Education, 22*, 289–303. https://doi.org/10.1080/0260293970220303

Thornton, R. L., Powe, N. R., Roter, D., & Cooper, L. A. (2011). Patient-physician social concordance, medical visit communication and patients' perceptions of health care quality. *Patient Education and Counseling, 85*(3), e201-e208. https://doi.org/10.1016/j.pec.2011.07.015

US Department of Health and Human Services. (2010). *Healthy People 2020: An opportunity to address the societal determinants of health in the United States.* Office of Disease Prevention and Health Promotion, Secretary's Advisory Committee on Health Promotion and Disease Prevention Objectives for 2020. https://www.cdc.gov/nchs/healthy_people/hp2020.htm

US Department of Health and Human Services. (2011). *Reflecting America's population. Diversifying a competent health care workforce for the 21ˢᵗ century. A statement of principles and recommendations.* Office of Minority Health, Advisory Committee on Minority Health. https://cg-d102dd1b-a880-440b-9eae-e2445148aee9.s3.us-gov-west-1.amazonaws.com/s3fs-public/documents/FinalACMHWorkforceReport.pdf

Vespa, J., Medina L., & Armstrong, D. M. (2020). *Demographic turning points for the United States: Population projections for 2020 to 2060.* Current Population Reports (P25-1144). https://www.census.gov/content/dam/Census/library/publications/2020/demo/p25-1144.pdf

Wilbur, K., Snyder, C., Essary, A. C., Swapna, R., Will, K. K., & Saxon, M. (2020). Developing workforce diversity in the health professions: A social justice perspective. *Health Professions Education, 6*(2), 222-229. https://doi.org/10.1016/j.hpe.2020.01.002

Understanding the Experiences of Black Medical Students

Katherine D. Daly, MA, PhD[1], Heather C. Rashal, MA[1], Matthew P. Abrams, MD[1], Melodie P. Noel, MD[1], D' Shaun Adams, MD[1], Matthew Parkin, BS[2], Patrick Kroenung, MD[1]

Author Affiliations: [1]University of Central Florida College of Medicine, Orlando, FL; [2]Herbert Wertheim College of Medicine, Florida International University, Miami, FL

Corresponding Author: Katherine Daly, Department of Clinical Sciences, University of Central Florida College of Medicine, 6850 Lake Nona Blvd, Orlando, FL, 32827 (katherine.daly@ucf.edu)

ABSTRACT

Adequate numbers of Black physicians are necessary to reduce the health disparities and inequities that impair US patient care. However, while comprising 12–14% of the US population, Black students represent only 6% of Liaison Committee on Medical Education (LCME)-accredited medical school enrollees. Medical schools may aim to recruit a diverse student body, to train culturally sensitive/competent clinicians, and to create supportive learning environments, but they lack the feedback to guide these efforts. This study captures the unique experiences of 15 Black students at allopathic medical schools in Florida to derive useful insights into how to better support them. It uses a qualitative approach, based on grounded theory, to analyze responses to anonymous surveys. The 13 questions addressed such topics as access, professional identity formation, preclinical and clerkship curricula, and barriers to, and facilitators of, success. Analysis identified 56 themes. Findings show that Black medical students rely on longstanding motivations, personal resilience, and solidarity with other underrepresented staff and faculty to navigate an educational experience characterized by disconnection, limited representation and mentorship, discrimination, and financial barriers.

Keywords: ▪ Diversity ▪ Black ▪ Medical School ▪ Learning Environment

J Best Pract Health Prof Divers, (Spring, 2024), 17(1), 55–66.
ISBN 2745-2843 © Winston-Salem State University

Authors' Note: We thank the students and institutions participating in this qualitative study and sharing their valuable perspectives with us.

INTRODUCTION

US medical schools are challenged to recruit a diverse body of students who will enhance the physician workforce and be responsive to the healthcare needs of an ever-changing society. Students from backgrounds underrepresented in medicine face barriers before they even apply to medical schools. They often have limited access to financial and other resources that increase competitiveness, such as standardized test preparation and guidance about the application process. Pipeline programs help (Lucey & Saquil, 2020), but without sufficient mentoring from Black role-models, they cannot overcome all systemic barriers.

The challenges escalate after acceptance. Medical students are expected to succeed through strenuous preclinical and clinical training. Academic demands affect most students' wellbeing, and underrepresentation only exacerbates them (Hardeman et al., 2015; Perry et al., 2015). Although medical schools have support systems for students to report on their classroom and clinical experiences, including racism, mistreatment, and microaggressions, students must trust that action will be taken and not against them. Lack of Black faculty and staff impedes them from establishing a network of social support and mentorship.

According to the US Census Bureau (2020), 12–14% of the national population is Black, yet Blacks comprise only 6% of the student body at LCME-accredited medical schools, including historically Black colleges and universities (HBCUs) (Poole, Jordan, & Bostwick, 2020).

This qualitative study focuses on the experiences of Black students at Florida medical schools. The overall aim is to provide medical schools with the information needed to increase the recruitment, matriculation, and success of Black medical students.

METHODS

Participant Recruitment

This qualitative, cross-sectional study was conducted at the University of Central Florida College of Medicine (UCF COM). A recruitment email with a Qualtrics survey was sent to allopathic medical schools across Florida. The recruitment materials were also circulated to the regional Student National Medical Association (SNMA) email list and regional channels for communication between Black medical students.

Eligibility criteria included being at least 18 years of age, enrolled as a medical student, and self-identifying as Black. UCF's Institutional Review Board (IRB) deemed the study exempt (IRB reference: STUDY00003276). Data were collected from August to October in 2021.

Survey Instrument

The research team designed a 14-item survey (see Appendix 1; question 14 was ultimately dropped from the analysis) to assess students' access to medical education and their experience of the curriculum, health disparities, and race's impact on their social life and professional identity formation. The survey included demographic questions about ethnicity, age, year in medical school, gender, sexual orientation, native country, languages spoken, and income. They were selected, drafted, and refined following a review of the literature on African American medical student experiences and team discussion. Most questions were designed to be open-ended and nondirective.

Grounded Theory Data Analysis Procedure

Grounded theory analysis was used to identify themes in the students' survey responses (Glaser et al., 2013). Complex, flexible, and systematic, grounded theory was originally developed to explore thematic elements in multifaceted responses that may be difficult to quantify (Chun Tie, Birks, & Francis, 2019). It is ideal for research focused on human experiences as it allows investigators to examine rich qualitative data related to the research questions in a nuanced way.

Grounded theory analysis requires three progressive coding levels: open, axial, and selective (Noble & Mitchell, 2016). Open code is the first level and can include a word, sentence, or partial sentence that points to a category. Axial coding enables researchers to connect these categories into broader themes (Chun Tie, Birks, & Francis, 2019). Selective coding builds a "grounded theory" from the themes. None of these codes is specified before the text analysis but emerge from reading the responses.

The research team met weekly on four separate occasions to identify and sort themes in the de-identified responses to each question. First, all texts were coded and reviewed for patterns across the data set. Three to four members independently identified open codes over several iterations to enable the emergence of novel themes and came together to confirm reliability. The senior author (KD) resolved any conflicts. At subsequent meetings, the team sorted the open codes into axial themes relevant to the experiences of Black medical students. The study focuses on the open and axial codes rather than identifying a summative grounded theory, which is optional (Chun Tie, Birks, & Francis, 2019).

Research Team and Potential Biases

The investigative team was made up of five medical students, one staff member, and one faculty member. It was balanced in terms of gender (three women, four men). Of the students, three identified as Black. The others have background and training in health equity. The faculty member is a licensed psychologist, an associate professor who serves as Director of Counseling and Wellness Services at UCF COM. The staff member is a licensed mental health counselor who treats medical students. The research team thus gathered the diverse perspectives of expert, learner, educator, and clinician.

RESULTS

In response to the 13 unique survey questions (question 14 was omitted from the data analysis), 56 axial themes emerged. Table 1 provides a detailed description of each. Here, we summarize the findings and their relationship to the literature.

When describing perceived barriers, students cited the lack of mentorship resulting from poor representation of Black faculty, consistent with studies in which both academic faculty and trainees from underrepresented backgrounds report feelings of isolation (Soliman et al., 2019). Comments supported connecting with minority peers and forming stronger connections with people of similar backgrounds. When asked if race had an impact on their sense of connection with faculty, participants expressed the desire for more minority faculty. Our findings are consistent with the literature depicting a lack of connection with staff when diversity is limited (Morrison, Machado, & Blackburn, 2019).

Overall, respondents identified a need for improvement in addressing race-related topics during the preclinical curriculum. These topics were covered sporadically in isolated lectures that relied heavily on stereotypes. A lack of engagement was noted, and meaningful conversations were limited, rushed, or cut short. Still, students felt schools were making more effort in response to the Black Lives Matter movement. In a study of the clerkship years (White & Ojugbele, 2019), most respondents stated that race-related issues in healthcare are not adequately addressed.

Moreover, the Association of American Medical Colleges Curriculum Inventory (AAMC CI) Report on Racial Disparities found that the vast majority of accredited US medical schools that have integrated racial healthcare disparities into their curriculum have done so in the preclinical years, although clinical settings are where these issues predominate (Brooks, Rougas, & George, 2016). Some students noticed a distinction in care during clinical rotations, specifically citing blood pressure treatment. Amutah et al. (2021) determined that the differential use of antihypertensives for African American patients is an example of medical schools' misrepresentation of race-based clinical guidelines.

Again, during the preclinical or clerkship years, 40% of respondents reported experiencing or witnessing racism/discrimination at their medical school. One student felt positive about the school's response and received support. Others felt hesitant to report. Some felt discomfort in making a report due to a sense its critique was dismissed or fear of being targeted and would rather talk to the individual. If the administration took action, respondents perceived the changes as mild progress that would benefit future cohorts. This study shows that the highest leadership may believe they are doing everything possible to address these problems, but students are skeptical.

In addition to instilling medical knowledge and clinical skills, medical school is critical for professional identity development, as undergraduate students transition to resident physicians (Goldie, 2012). Our study gathered a heterogenous set of experiences, ranging from no problems, to feeling conflicted, to having difficulty in integrating professional and personal identity. The need to strike a balance highlights a psychosocial stressor unique to the Black experience; the literature attests that higher degrees of racial identification increase anxiety and depression throughout medical school. Our respondents highlighted a feeling of obligation to advocacy and helping underrepresented patients. Cultural sensitivity, familiarity, and a welcoming atmosphere were described as influencing the medical school experience.

Study participants also reported strategies for success, which we categorize as (a) interpersonal support; (b) institutional support; and (c) self-reliance. Interpersonal support included building relationships with peers and faculty, particularly from minority backgrounds. Institutional support included academic assistance from organizations like SNMA and diversity, equity, and inclusion (DEI) departments. At the individual level, respondents referenced self-reliance, grit, authenticity, and determination to pave their own way through medical school.

We asked participants to share what they believe would make medical education more accessible to future Black students. The themes gathered included financial assistance, mentorship, increased access to early educational and research opportunities, and increasing Black representation among faculty.

DISCUSSION

This study captures the unique experiences of Black students at Florida medical schools. It aims to address the paucity of literature on the experiences and barriers these students face. Many medical schools have a sincere desire to recruit a diverse student body, train culturally sensitive/competent clinicians, and create a healthy and supportive learning environment. However, without adequate knowledge and feedback about what may be hindering these aspirations, they do not have the information necessary to make effective changes.

Based on our study's findings, a conceptual framework emerges. Black students rely on strong motivations, personal resilience, and solidarity with other underrepresented students and faculty

Table 1: Primary Themes and Subthemes

Survey Questions	Axial Thems
1. What led you to pursue medical education?	• Helping my community, helping others, helping those in need • Previous shadowing/medical experience • Personal experience with illness (family, friend, or self) • Health disparities, social injustice • Interest in science • Financial security
2. What are the strengths you bring to medicine?	• Empathy and compassion • Passion for service/helping/humanitarian/invested in people • Resilience, determination, hard-working • Cultural competence • Experience as a minority, a different perspective • Ability to connect with patients
3. What are the barriers or challenges you have experienced as a Black medical student?	• Lack of access/opportunities, knowledge, exposure (inequity in access), resources (financial), board preparation, shadowing • Fewer personal connections in medicine among family and friends; no inside knowledge of the process • Lack of mentorship, representation (faculty and physicians), hard to fit in • Unsupportive advisors, microaggressions, imposter syndrome
4. What helped you to be successful as a Black medical student?	• Interpersonal support (friends, peers, mentors, minority faculty, parents) • Structure in studying and schedule; sticking to plan; lifestyle and coping skills • Individualism/grit – paved my own way, doing my own research, using my own resources • Institutional support (SNMA, DEI, academic enrichment, tutoring. and academic advising)

5. What advice would you give to an incoming medical student who identifies as Black?	• Preserve confidence/maintain sense of self/authenticity
	• Imposter syndrome (combatting these feelings – you are capable, smart, deserving)
	• Mentorship
	• Don't be afraid to ask for help/Seek help
	• Finding community
	   • Support system
	   • Friends/peers
	   • Family

6. **Are there systematic changes that you think would make medical education more accessible to Black students?**	• Finances (MCAT, application fees, scoring fees) • Mentorship (every applicant had a mentor, connections) • Educational resources/access to early education/research/pipeline • Representation (hiring more minority faculty – make the journey seem more attainable)
7. **What has your experience been of forming a professional identity during medical school? How did you integrate your professional identity with other aspects of your identity development?**	• Authenticity (Stay true to self; "Professionalism doesn't mean abandoning your identity") • Advocacy (helping underrepresented patients; feeling the need to advocate) • Mentorship (find a mentor I identify with) • The learning environment of the medical school can set the tone (welcoming, familiar, stress cultural sensitivity in curriculum) • Heterogeneous experiences with regard to professional identity integration • Ranges from no problem, conflicted, difficulty
8. **Did your race have any impact on your social life and sense of connectedness with peers as a medical student?**	• All but one respondent identified an impact of race on connections – being open leads to good connections • Easier to bond/connect with people who are racially/ethnically similar (e.g., Haitian, Caribbean) • "Gravitate toward those who look like me" • Easier to connect with minority peers • Cultural events are a good way to connect
9. **Did your race have any impact on your sense of connectedness with faculty and staff at your medical school?**	• Yes, connection easier with minority faculty and staff ("background is an obvious thing to connect with someone on"; "made some relationships with five Black/Caribbean faculty members") • Connection is lacking when staff/faculty lack diversity ("felt less connected to faculty since I did not look like them"; "some staff ignored me or brushed me off") • Wish there were more minority faculty

(Continued)

Survey Questions	Axial Thems
10. Do you feel your medical school adequately addresses race and race-related topics in healthcare (such as health disparities, cultural competency) during the preclinical curriculum? Are these topics covered in isolated lectures/sessions or integrated throughout the preclinical curriculum?	• No, covered as isolated/sporadic/surface topics; heavy on stereotypes; need for improvement is consensus • Lack of engagement; ineffective ("fluff"); good conversations are limited, rushed, cut short
11. Do you feel your medical school adequately addresses race and race-related issues in healthcare (such as health disparities, cultural competency) during clerkship? Are these topics covered in isolated lectures/sessions or integrated throughout the clinical experience?	• Mostly "no" ("the effects of race in healthcare are not integrated in any formal way during the clerkship years") • Stereotypes, isolated coverage, surface level rather than deep • Noticing distinction in care on clinical rotation (e.g., blood pressure treatment)
12. Have you experienced or witnessed racism or discrimination at your medical school during preclinical or clerkship years? If so, would you feel comfortable reporting your concerns about lack of safety or mistreatment to an administrator at your medical school?	• 40% of respondents "yes"; 60% "no" • Of four who experienced racism, one felt positive about the response and received support; the other three felt hesitant to report and were not entirely comfortable making a report (reasons: felt dismissed; would rather talk to someone; fear of being targeted) • Some indicated that their school takes mistreatment/racism seriously (even if the student didn't experience it directly)
13. In situations where you've expressed concerns about race-related issues, such as mistreatment, discrimination, or lack of diversity and inclusion, did you feel administrators responded to your concerns effectively and took appropriate action?	• 3 respondents "yes"; 4 "no" • Dismissiveness ("foot-dragging", "met with action", "concern but not much action"; "I was completely ignored by my campus dean") • In cases where action is taken, it is viewed as "mild progress" that benefits future classes • Disconnect between student and administrators

to navigate an educational experience characterized by alienation, limited representation and mentorship, discrimination, and financial barriers. The axial themes that emerged from our survey questions provide rich data.

The study is limited by the small sample (n = 15). Although 34 students accessed the survey, some did not meet eligibility requirements, and some experienced technical difficulties, rendering survey data incomplete. Future studies should enlarge the sample to the national level and compare our survey findings from HBCUs to other medical schools. Last, the survey questions may complement existing measures (M2 and graduation questionnaires) that yield more insights into the perspectives of Black medical students to promote more inclusive learning environments.

REFERENCES

Amutah, C., Greenidge, K., Mante, A., et al. (2021). Misrepresenting race: The role of medical schools inpropagating physician bias. *New England Journal of Medicine, 384*(9), 872–878. https://doi.org/10.1056/NEJMms2025768

Brooks, K. C., Rougas, S., & George, P. (2016). When race matters on the wards: Talking about racial health disparities and racism in the clinical setting. *MedEdPORTAL, 12*, 10523. https://doi.org/10.15766/mep_2374-8265.10523

Chun Tie, Y., Birks, M., & Francis, K. (2019). Grounded theory research: A design framework for novice researchers. *SAGE Open Medicine, 7*, 2050312118822927. https://doi.org/10.1177/2050312118822927

Glaser, B., Walsh, I., Bailyn, L., Fernandez, W., Holton, J. A., & Levina, N. (2013). Whatgrounded theory is.... *Academy of Management Proceedings, 2013*(1). https://doi.org/10.5465/ambpp.2013.11290symposium

Goldie, J. (2012). The formation of professional identity in medical students: Considerations for educators. *Medical Teacher, 34*(9), e641–648. https://doi.org/10.3109/0142159x.2012.687476

Hardeman, R. R., Perry, S. P., Phelan, S. M., Przedworski, J. M., Burgess, D. J., & van Ryn, M. (2016). Racial identity and mental well-being: The experience of African American medical students. A report from the Medical Student CHANGE study. *Journal of Racial and Ethnic Health Disparities, 3*(2), 250–258. https://doi.org/10.1007/s40615-015-0136-5

Lucey, C. R., & Saguil, A. (2020). The consequences of structural racism on MCAT scores and medical school admissions: The past is prologue. *Academic Medicine, 95*(3), 351–356. https://doi.org/10.1097/ACM.0000000000002939

Morrison, N., Machado, M., & Blackburn, C. (2019). Student perspectives on barriers to performance for black and minority ethnic graduate-entry medical students: A qualitative study in a West Midlands medical school. *BMJ Open, 9*(11), e032493. https://doi.org/10.1136 /bmjopen-2019-032493

Noble, H., & Mitchell, G. (2016). What is grounded theory? *Evidence-Based Nursing, 19*(2), 34–35. https://doi.org/10.1136/eb-2016-102306

Perry, S. P., Hardeman, R., Burke, S. E., Cunningham, B., Burgess, D. J., & van Ryn M. (2016). The impact of everyday discrimination and racial identity centrality on African American medical student well-being. A report from the Medical Student CHANGE study. *Journal of Racial and Ethnic Health Disparities, 3*(3), 519–526. https://doi.org/10.1007 /s40615-015-0170-3

Poole, K. G. Jr., Jordan, B. L., & Bostwick, J. M. (2020). Mission drift: Are medical school admissions committees missing the mark on diversity? *Academic Medicine, 95*(3), 357–360. https://doi.org/10.1097/ACM.0000000000003006

Soliman, Y. S., Rzepecki, A. K., Guzman, A. K., Williams, R. F., Cohen, S. R., Ciocon, D., & Halverstam, C. (2019). Understanding perceived barriers of minority medical students pursuing a career in dermatology. *JAMA Dermatology, 155*(2), 252–254. https://doi .org/10.1001/jamadermatol.2018.4813

US Census Bureau. (2021). *2020 census illuminates racial and ethnic composition of the country.* https://www.census.gov.

White, S., & Ojugbele, O. (2019). Addressing racial disparities in medical education. *AAMC Curriculum in Context, 6*(2).

APPENDIX A

A STUDY OF THE EXPERIENCES OF AFRICAN AMERICAN AND BLACK MEDICAL STUDENTS

Instructions: The following questions aim to highlight the unique experiences of African American and Black medical students. Thank you for taking the time to respond. All responses will be **anonymous** and **de-identified** (including institution information associated with specific responses). Thank you!

Demographics

1. What is your age? ____
2. What year are you in medical school? ____
3. How would you describe yourself in terms of gender (e.g., man, woman, non-binary, trans man, etc.)? _____
4. How would you describe your sexual orientation? _____
5. Do you identify as Black and/or African American? Yes or No
6. Using your own words, how would you describe your ethnicity? _____ (e.g., Nigerian, Haitian, Jamaican American, Multiracial, Hispanic, etc.)
7. Were you born in the United States? Yes or No
8. If you emigrated to the U.S., where did you emigrate from and at what age? _____
9. Is English your native language? Yes or No If no, what is your native language? _____
10. When considering your family's household income, what range is most accurate?
    Less than $25,000
    $25,000 to $49,999
    $50,000 to $74,999
    $75,000 to $99,999
    $100,000 to $149,999
    $150,000 to $199,999
    $200,000 or more

Survey Questions

1. What led you to pursue medical education?
2. What are the strengths you bring to medicine?

3. What are the barriers or challenges you have experienced as an AA/Black medical student?
4. What helped you to be successful as an AA/Black medical student?
5. What advice would you give to an incoming medical student who identifies as AA/Black?
6. Are there systematic changes that you think would make medical education more accessible to AA/Black students? If so, please feel free to elaborate.
7. What has your experience been of forming a professional identity during medical school? How did you integrate your professional identity with other aspects of your identity development (i.e., cultural)?
8. Did your race have any impact on your social life and sense of connectedness with peers as a medical student? If so, in what ways?
9. Did your race have any impact on your sense of connectedness with faculty and staff at your medical school?
10. Do you feel your medical school adequately addresses race and race-related topics in healthcare (such as health disparities, cultural competency) during the pre-clinical curriculum? Are these topics covered in isolated lectures/sessions or integrated throughout the *pre-clinical* curriculum? Please feel free to elaborate.
11. Do you feel your medical school adequately addresses race and race-related issues in healthcare (such as health disparities, cultural competency) during clerkship? Are these topics covered in isolated lectures/sessions or integrated throughout the *clinical* experience? Please feel free to elaborate.
12. Have you experienced or witnessed racism or discrimination at your medical school during pre-clinical or clerkship years? If you did experience this, would you feel comfortable reporting your concerns about lack of safety or mistreatment to an administrator at your medical school?
13. In situations where you've expressed concerns about race-related issues, such as mistreatment, discrimination, or lack of diversity and inclusion, did you feel administrators responded to your concerns effectively and took appropriate action?
14. If you do not feel the questions fully capture your experience as an AA/Black medical student or wish to add anything, we encourage you to elaborate about your experience in the space below.

The Wake Forest University School of Medicine Postbaccalaureate Research and Education Program (PREP): A Stepping Stone to Matriculation and Success in Biomedical Science Graduate Programs

Debra I. Diz, PhD[1], Shea Gilliam-Davis, PhD[1], TanYa M. Gwathmey, PhD, MS[1]

Author Affiliations: [1]Department of Surgery - Hypertension; Cardiovascular Sciences Center, Wake Forest University School of Medicine, Winston-Salem, NC

Corresponding Author: TanYa M. Gwathmey, Hypertension and Vascular Research Center, Cardiovascular Sciences Center, Wake Forest University School of Medicine, 575 N. Patterson Avenue, Suite 340, Winston-Salem, NC, 27157 (tgwathme@wakehealth.edu)

ABSTRACT

Despite two decades of concerted efforts to increase the diversity of the biomedical sciences workforce, distinct populations remain poorly represented: Blacks, Latinos, Pacific Islanders, Native Americans, first-generation college students, and individuals with disabilities or from disadvantaged backgrounds. With grant support from the National Institute of General Medical Sciences (NIGMS), Wake Forest University School of Medicine (WFUSM) developed the Postbaccalaureate Research and Education Program (PREP) to facilitate their entry into biomedical sciences graduate programs. From 2001–2017, 80 students participated in a 1–2-year research-intensive internship simulating graduate school. As a result, 96% applied to PhD or MD/PhD programs; 92% entered PhD or other advanced degree programs, with 92% retention. These outcomes demonstrate the efficacy of a graduate-level preparatory program for diversifying the biomedical sciences workforce.

Keywords: ▪ Biomedical Sciences ▪ Diversity ▪ Education ▪ Post-Baccalaureate ▪ Underrepresented

J Best Pract Health Prof Divers (Spring, 2024), 17(1), 67–71.
ISBN 2745-2843 © Winston-Salem State University

Authors' Note: The authors gratefully acknowledge the National Institute of General Medical Sciences R25 grant (#GM064249) for programmatic support.

INTRODUCTION

Despite long-term efforts, certain groups remain poorly represented in science, technology, engineering, and math (STEM) careers. The number of Blacks, Latinos, Native Americans, Pacific Islanders, first-generation college students, and individuals with disabilities or from disadvantaged backgrounds in these fields hardly reflects their percentage of the overall US population (NIGMS, 2016). To address this inequity in healthcare settings and its consequential contribution to health disparities (Cohen, Gabriel, & Terrell, 2002), the National Institute of General Medical Sciences (NIGMS) promoted initiatives to increase diversity. The Wake Forest University School of Medicine (WFUSM) Postbaccalaureate Research and Education Program (PREP; R25 GM064249) was among the first funded in 2001.

PREP's goal is to increase diversity in the biomedical sciences workforce by increasing the entry and retention of underrepresented minorities in PhD programs both nationally and internally (Hall, Mann, & Bender, 2015). It provides minority students who earned a baccalaureate degree (BA, BS) in the prior 36 months with 1–2 years of intensive research experiences, professional skills training, career guidance, and Graduate Record Examinations (GRE) preparation to enhance the likelihood of acceptance into, and successful completion of, PhD programs. The experience gained is crucial to counterbalance the effect of lower GRE scores, well-documented among underrepresented groups, noting that such scores do not predict success in completing the PhD or achieving a successful research career (Hall, O'Connell, & Cook, 2017). This paper updates outcomes since our earlier report (Gwathmey, Tallant, Howlett, & Diz, 2016).

METHODS AND RESULTS

PREP components include: 1) full-time engagement in a biomedical research project; 2) graduate-level coursework; 3) a GRE preparation course; 4) professional skills development, including writing and presentation; and 5) individual development plans (IDPs), drafted by the trainee in concert with program directors and research mentors, to identify personal academic goals and objectives, strategies to achieve success, and metrics for accountability. PREP Scholars identify research mentors from a large cadre of established scientists conducting research in their field of interest. They choose career mentors who align with their long-term professional development and career interests.

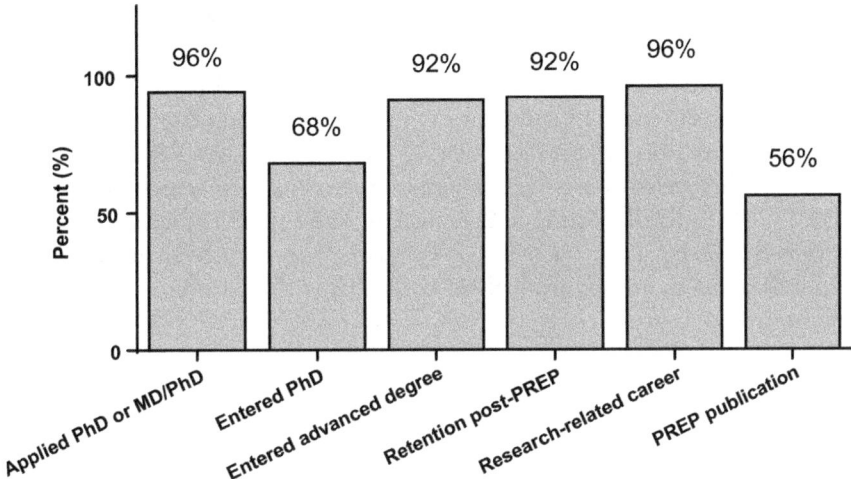

Figure 1: Summary Statistics for PREP.

Distribution of outcomes for participants in the Postbaccalaureate Research and Education Program (PREP). The percentage of those who entered advanced degree programs (92%) approaches the percentage applying to PhD or MD/PhD programs. The percentage of those entering PhD programs is also included in the advanced degree values and represents the majority of advanced degrees.

Scholars enroll in coursework reflecting their goals and academic needs. They also take the required graduate courses in scientific integrity, ethics, and responsible conduct of research and a course that explores their many career options after PhD training. Each year ends with a research symposium at which the scholars present their findings to the institutional community, including their peers in the program, its directors and faculty, research and career mentors and their research teams, and graduate school admissions faculty. Families are invited to provide support and to encourage progression and pursuit of biomedical science careers.

PREP's administrative home is the Hypertension and Vascular Research Center in the Department of Surgery. Program participants receive a salary similar to a graduate student's stipend or that of first-year technical staff. The grant pays tuition costs and for travel to scientific and diversity-focused meetings. From 2001–2017, 80 scholars completed the program. Approximately 75% were African American; 20% Hispanic; 2% Asian/Pacific Islander; and 1% Native American. Their GPAs averaged 3.1 on a 4-point scale, illustrating the selection of students who may require PREP training to improve their chance of admission into advanced degree programs.

Figure 1 shows that 96% of participants applied to PhD or MD/PhD programs. Overall, 92% entered advanced degree programs: 68% entered a PhD program; 11% pursued health professional degrees; and 41% Master's degrees, both terminal and preceding entry into a PhD program. Of those who entered PhD programs, ~33% pursued their degree in WFU biomedical sciences programs. Retention in post-PREP degree programs averages 92%, with 94% retention at WFU. Note that their retention rate is well above the national averages reported at an earlier stage for NIGMS PREPs (Hall, Mann, & Bender, 2015) and the 75% reported for the biomedical sciences (Sowell, Zhang, Redd, & King, 2008). An impressive 56% of PREP scholars were authors on publications stemming from their work during the program, and ~96% remain in science-related careers.

CONCLUSION

From 2001–2017, WFUSM PREP added 77 students from underrepresented minority groups to work in the biomedical sciences. Most entered a PhD program, and their retention in PhD and other advanced degree programs is outstanding (>90%). While they gained admission into graduate programs nationwide, they have significantly increased diversity in WFU Biomedical Sciences programs: ~33% remained at WFU for their PhD training. Furthermore, their retention in research and research-related careers is exceptionally high (~96%). These indices of success attest a supportive environment, generating the self-efficacy and persistence necessary to complete advanced degrees (Estrada et al., 2016; Hurtado et al., 2011 McGee, Saran, & Krulwich, 2012). These outcomes are consistent with our earlier reports; participants in both PREP and our long-standing summer program have sustained a strong upward trajectory for diversifying the biomedical science workforce (Gwathmey, Tallant, Howlett, & Diz, 2016).

REFERENCES

Cohen, J. J., Gabriel, B. A., & Terrell, C. (2002). The case for diversity in the health care workforce. *Health Affairs, 21*(5), 90–102. https://doi.org/10.1377/hlthaff.21.5.90

Estrada, M., Burnett, M., Campbell, A. G., Denetclaw, W. F., Gutiérrez, C. G., Hurtado, S., John, G. H., Matsui, J., McGee, R., Okpodu, C. M., Robinson, T. J., Summers, M. F., Werner-Washburne, M., & Zavala, M. (2017). Improving underrepresented minority student persistence in STEM. *CBE Life Sciences Education, 15*, es5. https://doi.org/10.1187/cbe.16-01-0038

Gwathmey, T. M., Tallant, E. A., Howlett, A. C., & Diz, D. I. (2016). Programs to recruit and retain a more diverse workforce in biomedical sciences research. *Journal of Best Practices in Health Professions Diversity, 9*(1), 1188–1194. https://www.jstor.org/stable/26554246

Hall, A., Mann, J., & Bender, M. (2015). 2015 analysis of outcomes for the NIGMS postbaccalaureate research education program. https://www.nigms.nih.gov/News/reports/Documents/PREP-outcomes-report.pdf

Hall, J. D., O'Connell, A. B., & Cook, J. G. (2017). Predictors of student productivity in biomedical graduate school applications. *PLoS ONE, 12*(1), e0169121. https://doi.org/10.1371/journal.pone.016912

Hurtado, S., Eagan, M. K., Tran, M. C., Newman, C. B., Chang, M. J., & Velasco, P. (2011). "We do science here": Underrepresented students' interactions with faculty in different college contexts. *Journal of Social Issues, 67*(3), 553–579. https://doi.org/10.1111/j.1540-4560.2011.01714.x

McGee Jr, R., Saran, S., & Krulwich, T. A. (2012). Diversity in the biomedical research workforce: Developing talent. *Mount Sinai Journal of Medicine, 79*(3), 397–411. https://doi.org/10.1002/msj.21310

National Institute of General Medical Sciences (NIGMS). (2016, July 15). *Enhancing diversity in training programs.* https://www.nigms.nih.gov/Training/Diversity/Pages/Approaches.aspx

Sowell R., Zhang T., Redd, K., & King, M. F. (2008). *Ph.D. completion and attrition: Analysis of baseline program data from the Ph.D. completion project.* Council of Graduate Schools. http://www.phdcompletion.org/quantitative/book1_quant.asp

Recruiting and Retaining Diverse Nursing Faculty

Dennis Sherrod EdD, RN[1], Cecil Holland, EdD, PhD, RN[1]

Author Affiliations: [1]Division of Nursing, Winston-Salem State University, Winston-Salem, NC

Corresponding Author: Dennis Sherrod, Division of Nursing, Winston-Salem State University, 601 S. Martin Luther King, Jr. Drive, Winston-Salem, NC (sherrodd@wssu.edu)

INTRODUCTION

Demand for registered nurses and advanced practice nurses is growing. The US Bureau of Labor Statistics estimates that from 2021–2031, demand for registered nurses grew 6% (2022a) and for nurse practitioners 40% (2022b). Factors fueling this trend include increased preventive care; increasing incidence of chronic conditions, such as obesity, diabetes, and hypertension; and increasing demand for health services from baby-boomers.

To meet the pressing need, administrators of nursing-education programs can expect an increased focus on faculty recruitment and retention strategies. In 2022, faculty-position vacancy rates in US nursing-education programs ranged from 8.8% to 11% (Byrne et al., 2022). Common recruitment barriers include noncompetitive salaries (66.7%) and finding faculty who match the program specialty (59.2%) (Byrne et al., 2022). Short-term schemes, such as sign-on bonuses, can create a revolving door; applicants may be attracted but rapidly leave. Retention efforts can be the best recruitment strategy since creating a work culture that supports faculty often attracts others.

The need for greater diversity increases demand for recruitment and retention strategies that focus on diverse faculty. In recent years, the COVID-19 pandemic and prevalent health disparities have increased its urgency. We need more diverse nurse educators to reflect the population we serve more closely. The US Census Bureau (2022) estimates the population as 59.3% White, 18.9% Hispanic, 13.6% African American, 6.1% Asian, 2.9% multiracial, and 1.3% American Indian. About half of Americans identify as female (50.5%) or male (49.5%). US nurse educators are White (80.8%), African American (8.8%), Hispanic (3.2%), Asian (2.7%), multiracial (.6%), and American Indian (.4%) (National League for Nursing, 2017a) and predominately female (93.2%), with a small proportion of men (6.4%) (National League for Nursing, 2017b).

J Best Pract Health Prof Divers, (Spring, 2024), 17(1), 72–78.
ISBN 2745-2843 © Winston-Salem State University

The aim of this study is to identify recruitment and retention strategies that can help nursing-education programs to attract and retain a diverse faculty.

Diversity, Equity, and Inclusion (DEI)

Diversity includes differences in age, generational characteristics, ethnicity, race, gender identity, religion, sexual orientation, nationality, family background, country of origin, family status, socio-economic status, residence history (rural and/or urban), and other personal factors in an environment or an organization (Dehghanpour, 2022; Elliot, 2021). Nursing and nursing education can also address differences in educational preparation, specialty, work setting, and work experience.

Increasing DEI in the healthcare workforce helps to increase health access, improve the quality of care, stimulate innovation, and reduce health disparities (Cohen et al., 2002). Nursing and health sciences educational programs and work cultures that welcome everyone and embrace problem-solving processes that build on individual differences are more likely to achieve student learning outcomes and organizational goals. Administrative metrics and dashboards should include DEI goals to monitor performance, and monitoring faculty retention and promotions can drive DEI progress (Davenport et al., 2022).

Rather than requiring a new faculty member to "assimilate" to the work culture "norm", staff should inquire, listen, and embrace individual differences and preferences. The Golden Rule—"do unto others as you would have others do unto you"—is no longer acceptable. We must apply the "Platinum Rule" and do unto others what they would prefer. Bias, discrimination, and micro-aggressions are not acceptable in an inclusive workplace culture (Aysola et al., 2018; Davenport et al., 2021; Mateo & Williams, 2020; Mendoza et al., 2015).

Conversation and dialogue can be helpful in learning about differences and similarities. For example, nurse faculty share a goal: to help students achieve program learning outcomes. Some bring expertise in curriculum development; others, in teaching clinical skills; yet others, in conducting simulation scenarios. These differences combine to form a creative, more complete strategy. At the same time, a diverse faculty can promote more comfortable and effective teaching and learning relationships among diverse students. The goal is to create a sense of belonging for everyone.

Nurse Faculty Recruitment

Factors influencing recruitment and retention of nurse educators include the flexibility of the work schedule, job benefits, and salary (Arian, et al., 2018; Evans, 2013; Hand & Reid, 2022; Lee et al., 2017; Lo et al., 2019). Clinical supervision can impose a rigid work schedule since most nursing-education programs do not have personnel prepared to fill in when faculty call in sick or require a mental health day. Developing a pool of on-call adjunct faculty can assist with this challenge.

At least annually, nursing-education programs should ensure that their salaries and benefits are competitive. In many states, public university salaries can be accessed online, and such organizations as the American Association of Colleges of Nursing and the National League for Nurses often conduct faculty benefit and salary surveys. One approach nursing-education programs may find helpful is a "grow your own" faculty initiative, which invests funds to support tuition readmission and time off, so new faculty can attend classes and complete their Master's or doctoral degree.

Nursing-education programs should consider print, media, or online ads or branding campaigns upholding DEI as core values (Davenport et al., 2021). Institutional and departmental mission and vision statements should promote diversity and equity among faculty, students, and the community. Compared to big business, higher education has been slow to budget funding for ad campaigns, while hospitals and other healthcare settings now use them as a vital nurse-recruitment strategy. Higher education and nurse-education programs will have to follow suit to attract the expert faculty needed for specialty positions. To target advertising, a list of Master's and doctorally prepared nurses' email or home addresses can be acquired from the state Board of Nursing. Ads can be sent to the National Black Nurses Association or the National Association of Hispanic Nurses.

Faculty search committees must demonstrate diversity in rank, gender, race, specialty, and, where applicable, include staff and student representatives (Davenport et al., 2021; Graham, 2021). The number of members should be odd to prevent tie votes (Graham, 2021). Their training should review legal issues related to interviewing and hiring practices and discuss implicit bias. Davenport et al. (2021) recommend a holistic review of candidate applications to identify characteristics that the institution and educational program value. They suggest that committee members ask the same questions of each applicant and use a standardized scoring tool to rate responses.

Nurse Faculty Retention

New faculty should participate in institutional and departmental orientations. They should be assigned a faculty mentor to assist them in achieving personal and professional goals.

Factors that influence faculty job satisfaction and engagement include family-friendly policies, collaboration, consistency and approachability among departmental leaders, institutional leadership, and shared governance (Kippenbrock et al., 2022; Lee et al., 2017). Work roles, responsibilities, and requirements for advancement should be clearly defined in the job description and faculty handbook.

At least one faculty group should be charged with monitoring and making recommendations about work culture. Whether comprised of senior faculty, the full faculty, the committee should review policies to make sure they are inclusive and family-friendly. Policies for dealing with racism, discrimination, microaggressions, and other grievances must be in place. Professional development programs should help faculty and staff to recognize bias, and faculty and student handbooks should be reviewed to remove biased policies. The American Psychological Association Publication Manual (2020) recommends replacing gender-biased third-person pronouns, such as she, her, he, and his, with gender-neutral analogues, such as person, individual, they, them, and their.

Provide resources and support to assist nurse faculty in developing courses, teaching, and using technology in classroom and clinical settings. Winston-Salem State University's Center for Innovative and Transformative Instruction (CITI) is an "inclusive, supportive, and collaborative service for faculty, staff, and administrators to pursue innovation and transformation in higher education teaching and learning" (CITI, 2022, ¶1). Nurse faculty work with faculty across the university to develop courses and share successful implementation of technology in face-to-face and virtual classroom settings. Quality improvement should be part of everyday teaching and learning processes. Faculty should conduct an annual program evaluation with established benchmarks to monitor progress.

The nurse faculty work environment requires rigorous teaching, evaluation, and supervision of students as well as overseeing patient care in the clinical setting. Many times, nurses invest so much time providing care for others that they have little time to care for themselves. Self-care behaviors focusing on personal health, physical activity, nutrition, spiritual growth, interpersonal relations, mindful relaxation, and stress management promote resilience and help to prevent compassion fatigue and burnout (Rigdon & Winters, 2022; Zeb et al., 2022). Nursing-education programs must provide such resources as employee health clinics and flexible work schedules. Professional development opportunities can also focus on self-care and building a healthy work environment conducive to faculty, student, and patient well-being (Rigdon & Winters, 2022; Zeb et al., 2022).

CONCLUSION

The demand for registered nurses is greater now than at any time in history. Myriad factors contribute, including, but not limited to, longer lifetimes, leading to more chronic health conditions; greater consumer demand; and a national shortage of professional nurses. Nurse administrators must recognize the talent gaps across the profession and develop recruitment and retention strategies that mitigate the challenges of supply and demand.

A consistent challenge in academia is finding the right talent. As educational institutions are charged with increasing student enrollment in nursing programs, the difficulty is often attracting the right talent and the right fit. Intentional recruiting and retention efforts are essential to invite and retain this valuable human resource.

The faculty shortage in nursing schools across the country is real, and a large percentage of faculty are expected to retire over the next few years, with tremendous impact on nursing school enrollment capacity. Inadequate compensation contributes; nurse clinicians, often with less education, earn higher salaries than nurse academicians. More equitable compensation and flexible scheduling is a starting point for addressing the economic disparities.

Creating a culture of diversity, equity, and inclusion is critical, and it is simply the right thing to do. It must be embraced at all levels and visible in every aspect of the work: including strategic priorities, planning, holistic admissions, committee structures, evaluation, and faculty, staff, and student make-up. As we engage in DEI work, persistence is prudent. Professional nurses and nurse educators are perfectly positioned to champion and model DEI in recruiting and retention.

REFERENCES

American Psychological Association. (2020). *Publication manual of the American Psychological Association 2020: the official guide to APA style* (7th ed.). American Psychological Association.

Arian, M., Soleimani, M., & Oghazian, M. B. (2018). Job satisfaction and the factors affecting satisfaction in nurse educators: A systematic review. *Journal of Professional Nursing, 34*(5), 389–399. https://doi.org/10.1016/j.profnurs.2018.07.004

Aysola, J., Barg, F. K., Martinez, A.B., Kearney, M., Agesa, K., Carmona, C., & Higginbotham, E. (2018). Perceptions of factors associated with inclusive work and learning environments in health care organizations: A qualitative narrative analysis. *JAMA NetwOpen, 1*(4), e181003. https://doi.org/10.1001/jamanetworkopen.2018.1003

Byrne, C., Keyt, J., & Fang, D. (2022). *Special survey on vacant faculty positions for academic year 2022–2023.* https://www.aacnnursing.org/News-Information/Research-Data

Center for Innovative and Transformative Instruction (CITI). (2022). *Winston-Salem State University.* https://www.wssu.edu/administration/faculty-and-staff/citi/index.html

Cohen, J. J., Gabriel, B. A., & Terrell, C. (2002). The case for diversity in the health care workforce. *Health Affairs, 21*(5), 90–102. https://doi.org/10.1377/hlthaff.21.5.90

Davenport, D., Alvarez, A., Natesan, S., Caldwell, M. T., Gellegos, M., Landry, A., Parsons, M., & Gottlieb, M. (2021). Faculty recruitment, retention, and representation in leadership: An evidence-based guide to best practices for diversity, equity, and inclusion from the Council of Residency Directors in Emergency Medicine. *Western Journal of Emergency Medicine, 23*(1), 62–71. https://doi.org/10.5811/westjem.2021.8.53754

Deghanpour, M. (2022). Diversity, equity, and inclusion in health science education. *Radiologic Technology, 94*(2), 152–154.

Elliott, T. C. (2021). How do we move the needle? Building a framework for diversity, equity, and inclusion within graduate medical education. *Family Medicine, 53*(7), 556–558. https://doi.org/10.22454/FamMed.2021.199007

Evans, J. D. (2013). Factors influencing recruitment and retention of nurse educators reported by current nurse faculty. *Journal of Professional Nursing, 29*(1), 11–20. https://doi.org/10.1016/j.profnurs.2012.04.012

Graham, A. (2021). *Faculty for the future: Best practices for conducting faculty searches at WSSU. Manual 2021–22. Office of Faculty Affairs, Office of the Provost,* Winston-Salem State University. https://www.wssu.edu/about/office-of-the-provost/academic-and-administrative-units/faculty-affairs/_files/documents/faculty-recruitment-hiring-guidelines.pdf

Hand, M. C., & Reid, A. (2022). Men in nursing academia: Factors associated with recruitment and retention. *Nurse Educator, 47*(4), 246–251. https://doi.org/10.1097/NNE.0000000000001150

Kippenbrock, T., Rosen, C. C., & Emory, J. (2022). Job satisfaction among nursing faculty in Canada and the United States. *Journal of Nursing Education, 61*(11), 617–623. https://doi.org/10.3928/01484834-20220912-03

Laurencelle, F. L., Scanlan, J. M., & Brett, A. L. (2016). The meaning of being a nurse educator and nurse educators' attraction to academia: A phenomenological study. *Nurse Education Today, 39*, 135–140. https://doi.org/10.1016/j.nedt.2016.01.029

Lee, P., Miller, M. T., Kippenbrock, T. A., Rosen, C., & Emory, J. (2017). College nursing faculty job satisfaction and retention: A national perspective. *Journal of Professional Nursing, 33*(4), 261–266. https://doi.org/10.1016/j. profnurs.2017.01.001 PMID:28734484

Lo, M. C., Tolentino, J., Fazio, S. B., Vinciguerra, S., Amin, A. N., Dentino, A., Hingle, S. T., Palamara, K., Modak, I., Kisielewski, M., & Moriarty, J. P. (2020). Identifying solutions to ambulatory faculty recruitment, retention, and remuneration in graduate medical education: An AAIM position paper. *American Journal of Medicine, 133*(3), 386–394. https://doi.org/10.1016/j.amjmed.2019.11.001

Mateo, C. M., & Williams, D. R. (2020). More than words: A vision to address bias and reduce discrimination in the health professions learning environment. *Academic Medicine, 95*, S169-S177. https://doi.org/10.1097/ACM.0000000000003684

Mendoza, F. S., Walker, L. R., Stoll, B. J., Fuentes-Afflick, E., Geme, J. W., Cheng, T. L., Gonzalez del Rey, J. A., Harris, C. E., Rimsza, J. L., & Sectish, T. C. (2015). Diversity and inclusion training in pediatric departments. *Pediatrics, 135*(4), 707–713. https://doi.org/10.1542/peds.2014-1653

National League for Nursing. (2017a). *Disposition of full-time nurse educators by race-ethnicity.* https://www.nln.org/news/research-statistics/newsroomnursing-education-statistics/nurse-educator-demographics-2137b25c-7836-6c70-9642-ff00005f0421

National League for Nursing. (2017b). *Disposition of full-time nurse educators by gender.* https://www.nln.org/news/research-statistics/newsroomnursing-education-statistics/nurse-educator-demographics-2137b25c-7836-6c70-9642-ff00005f0421

Rigdon, K. L. & Winters, K. (2022). Relationships among self-care, compassion satisfaction, and compassion fatigue of nurses in community hospitals in the southeastern United

States. *International Journal of Human Caring, 26*(2), 83–91. https://doi.org/10.20467/HumanCaring-D-19-00036

US Bureau of Labor Statistics (2022a). *Occupational outlook handbook.* Registered nurses. https://www.bls.gov/ooh/healthcare/nurse-anesthetists-nurse-midwives-and-nurse-practitioners.htm

US Bureau of Labor Statistics (2022b). *Occupational outlook handbook.* Nurse anesthetists, nurse midwives, and nurse practitioners. https://www.bls.gov/ooh/healthcare/registered-nurses.htm

United States Census Bureau. (2022). *Quick facts: United States.* https://www.census.gov/quickfacts/fact/table/US/PST045222

Youngclaus, J., & Roskovensky, L. (2018). An updated look at the economic diversity of US medical students. *AAMC Analysis in Brief, 18*(5), 1–3. https://www.aamc.org/media/9596/download?attachment

Zeb, H., Arif, I., & Younas, A. (2022). Mindful self-care practice of nurses in acute care: A multisite cross-sectional survey. *Western Journal of Nursing Research, 44*(6), 540–547. https://doi.org/10.1177/0193945921100

So Hard to be a Ram: A Student Perspective

Taylor E. Daniels, MS, BA[1], Nia N. Battle, MPH, BA[1]

Author Affiliations: [1]Department of Exercise Physiology, Winston-Salem State University, Winston-Salem, NC

Corresponding Author: Taylor E. Daniels, Department of Exercise Physiology, Winston-Salem State University, 601 S. Martin Luther King, Jr Dr., Winston-Salem, NC (*Tedanie98@gmail.com*)

INTRODUCTION

Historically Black Colleges/Universities (HBCUs) clearly differ in many ways from Predominantly White Institutions (PWIs), from the offices that manage policies and financial stability to student engagement and campus culture. Students who attend HBCUs enjoy a tight-knit community that contributes to their success. For many Black students, the opportunity to be true to themselves and their cultural identity while pursuing their academic interests fosters a uniquely supportive learning environment.

Critics continue to question minority-serving institutions as they fight for their space in higher education. Some question the quality of the education, but HBCUs boast notable alumni, including Vice-President Kamala Harris, sports commentator Stephen A. Smith, and talk-show host Oprah Winfrey. Each university has its own history, but they are connected by a similar purpose: to elevate and educate Black students. Formerly Winston-Salem Teachers College, Winston-Salem State University (WSSU) contributes to the rich legacy of HBCUs.

The authors interviewed each other, and their responses are transcribed below. Each question was formulated to touch on different aspects of their academic journeys and to give them the space to express their honest opinions.

Why did you select your college or university?

Nia: *I selected Winston-Salem State University for multiple reasons. It was the only university that I attended open house events for. The alumni in my hometown, Goldsboro, North Carolina, were very influential and always were happy to show their RAM PRIDE! Due to originally being interested in Nursing, I was very*

J Best Pract Health Prof Divers, (Spring, 2024), 17(1), 79–83.
ISBN 2745-2843 © Winston-Salem State University

impressed at the ranking of the institution. I always wanted to attend a historically Black college or university; therefore, WSSU was the perfect match.

Taylor: *Like Nia, the alumni influence in our hometown of Goldsboro, North Carolina significantly impacted my decision to attend Winston-Salem State University. It was evident that they truly enjoyed the institution and the experiences they created while there as students. When I was thinking about applying to colleges, I did not have a dream school in mind, but when I stepped on the campus of WSSU, it felt like home. The university also offered me the opportunity to pursue my passions beyond the bounds of the classroom. I originally entered the school with a dream of continuing into their physical therapy (PT) program, because of its successful track record. I later changed my academic path and decided to focus on premedical education. WSSU also provided me with the opportunity to participate in intercollegiate athletics as a member of the Women's Basketball team.*

Do you think your grades are a good indication of your academic achievement?

Nia: *I would have to say yes and no. While at WSSU, I faced many challenges as I know others did around me. I would like to say that my grades in certain courses first showed what I actually enjoyed, truly understood, and what other factors were present during that time. To some, my grades were good, but to me, I know they could have been better. Though my grades did not meet my personal standards, I was still able to pursue and complete a graduate program after my time at WSSU.*

Taylor: *Fortunately, my grades are a very good representation of my academic achievement. I maintained strong academic credentials during my undergraduate career, and that trend continued into my graduate studies. While my grades are good, I am aware they are not the only marker of academic achievement. As a result, I have tried to add other experiences to my resume that develop me holistically as a student and individual.*

Have you completed any internships? What did you gain from the experience?

Nia: *Unfortunately, I did not participate in an internship during my undergraduate career. I actually became more interested in my public health minor than I thought I would. I decided that I wanted to obtain a Master's in public health; therefore, I began to look into opportunities that would help me with that goal. I began to work closely with my professor, Dr. Kineka J. Hull. Luckily, I was able to seek other opportunities outside of the university, such as volunteering and shadowing, to gain experience and enhance my knowledge in the area.*

Taylor: *While at WSSU, I completed an internship in the corporate office of a large grocery retailer during the summer between my junior and senior years. My summer project focused on how to make healthy eating achievable and budget friendly for all customers, especially those from low socioeconomic backgrounds. I realized the importance of community infrastructure, such as supermarkets, and the potential impact it could have on individual and communal outcomes. At this point in my academic journey, I decided I wanted to pursue a public health-oriented career in medicine to promote holistic wellness. I became interested in improving people's physical health in conjunction with their overall well-being. This opportunity allowed me to take the knowledge that I acquired from WSSU and translate it into real-world experience.*

What extracurricular activities have you participated in?

Nia: *The main extracurricular activity I participated in was employment. I worked all four years of my collegiate career except for one summer. During the summer that I was not able to find employment, I went to summer school for security. I was blessed to work as a resident advisor during my time at WSSU. Senior year, I decided to move off-campus. During this time I maintained two jobs. During all four years, I volunteered with various organizations/facilities on campus and around Winston-Salem, NC.*

Taylor: *During my time on campus, I played on the Women's Basketball team, while maintaining my place in the Simon Green Atkins Honor Society. I also became a member of the Gamma Lambda chapter of Alpha Kappa Alpha Sorority, Inc., and conducted undergraduate research. These experiences allowed me to become a well-rounded student and greatly contributed to my college experience.*

What was your biggest challenge as a student, and how did you handle it?

Nia: *My biggest challenge would have to be preparing for the things that would follow at the completion of my time at WSSU. I found that there weren't many skills taught tailored to life after graduation. As a 2020 graduate, finishing undergraduate studies during a pandemic has been both a blessing and a curse due to the many changes that were set in place for graduate programs and professional placement.*

Though I understand the seriousness and the impact that the pandemic has had upon the world, including WSSU (faculty/staff, students, etc.), I think we should also acknowledge the major role of career/professional development when trying to advance. I was fortunate to build relationships with certain professors who helped with this process. Some even being as simple as having a conversation that resulted in a learning experience or networking opportunity.

Taylor: *My biggest challenge while at WSSU was professional and academic development. I felt as if I lacked the necessary knowledge and resources needed to advance my career. This is part of the reason I took time to complete a Master's program before applying to medical school. WSSU offered me many opportunities, but there were disparities in access to resources when I compared my experiences to counterparts from other institutions. General guidance regarding applications, admissions, and other medical school logistics, such as costs, was hard to find.*

During my senior year, I joined a premedical association on campus, but it was not as beneficial as I would have hoped. This could have been attributed to the interference of the pandemic when my senior year ended abruptly. If it had not been for my helpful academic advisor, I would not have known about the graduate program I was accepted into at Wake Forest University. After being in my graduate program for a few months, there were simple things I wish I had previously known, such as the finances associated with applications and helpful Medical College Admission Test (MCAT) study tips.

What is your greatest strength as a student?

Nia: *I would say, my greatest strength as a student would have to be my resilience. Like others, I encountered a lot during my academic career. I have seen people give up or lack self-fulfillment due to challenges faced* *during the collegiate career. Developing a level of honesty and acceptance with yourself is important; it allows you to understand that it is all right if things didn't go as you may have originally planned. I am determined to keep going and believe that what is for me will be for me.*

Taylor: *I would say that my greatest strength as a student is my work ethic. I've continuously put in the time to be successful inside and outside of the classroom.*

How has your college experience prepared you for a career?

Nia: *My overall academic journey has prepared me. I quickly found out that it is not always about what you know but who you know. Obtaining a degree in exercise science helped me greatly, but it is not a terminal degree; therefore, I must obtain a higher level of education if I want to be a competitive candidate for a career with my degree. The combination of my degree, concentration (public health), and minor (psychology) has helped me greatly. It has allowed me to understand the application and use of various models and theories.*

Taylor: *During my time at WSSU, I learned the importance of perseverance and humility. I was challenged academically and professionally as I developed throughout my college career. Recognizing when I needed help and accepting it willingly propelled me to where I am today. It may seem simple, but these two lessons carried me through my schooling and contributed greatly to the success post-graduation.*

Action items/Next steps for the university:

Exercise Physiology Department:

The department should continue to educate and train students with academic rigor. It can prepare students who are interested in the many Exercise Physiology-related careers, while also exposing them to other occupations in healthcare. While Exercise Physiology is commonly used as a steppingstone to careers in physical therapy, athletic training, or academia, it can also be used as an avenue to jobs in medicine, occupational therapy, or nutrition. Diversifying the teaching staff to represent a greater variety of academic backgrounds could also be beneficial. It would encourage students to explore all of their career options as they navigate their collegiate journeys.

School of Allied Health Sciences:

A pre-health professions advisory committee that represents a variety of professional and academic backgrounds could provide an array of tools and insight students need to become successful. It would be a vital resource for career development, educational mapping, and financial planning for their future academic endeavors. At other institutions, such committees have proven to be extremely beneficial for students applying to a variety of professional programs. They provide support and helpful services, such as letters of recommendation, that may aid in a student's application processes and future success. A letter of recommendation from a committee can often replace the required letters from individual faculty members or employers that an applicant would otherwise have to gather for their professional school application. Securing the single recommendation letter allows students to focus on other important pieces of their applications. Ultimately, a pre-health committee would help students as they navigate from WSSU to professional programs.

CONCLUSION

WSSU continues to produce excellent students who succeed in all areas of their lives. The authors hope their personal guidance, advice, and suggestions can help the next generation of WSSU students. Students should pay forward the benefits of their education in acts of service, such as this manuscript. As proud alumnae, the authors are excited to envision a successful future for the university and its students.

REFERENCE

Doyle, A. (2019, December 4). Common college job interview questions and answers. *The Balance*. https://www.thebalancemoney.com/college-job-interview-questions-and-answers-2061193